The Vitamin B6 Book

by Ruth Adams
and
Frank Murray

Larchmont Books
New York

First printing: July, 1980

THE VITAMIN B6 BOOK

Copyright © Larchmont Books, 1980

ISBN 0-915962-30-6

Printed in the United States of America

LARCHMONT BOOKS
6 East 43rd Street
New York, N.Y. 10017
Tel., 212-949-0800

Contents

CHAPTER 1

The Importance of Pyridoxine (Vitamin B₆)

THE NUTRITIONAL IMPORTANCE of vitamin B_6—pyridoxine— has been recognized for a rather short time, considering that it was first isolated in 1934 by Dr. Paul György. It is known that the body has a continuous need for this vitamin, which must be met by the intake of vitamin B_6 from food or food supplements. So far there is no evidence that it can be manufactured by bacteria in the human intestinal tract, such as the case with biotin, another member of the B complex.

According to the Vitamin Information Bureau, Inc., New York, vitamin B_6 takes part in an amazing number of chemical reactions within the body. It serves mainly as a co-enzyme in various metabolic steps by which amino acids or building blocks of protein are synthesized, degraded or transformed from one to another. Therefore, the vitamin is needed for optimum utilization of dietary protein. It is also important for many other metabolic reactions, especially those involving lipids (fats) and carbohydrates.

"As a matter of fact," reports Otto A. Bessey, "there are probably few reactions of the amino acids in living organisms in which enzymes containing vitamin B_6 are not involved, hence the term 'amino acid metabolism vitamin.'"

It seems almost impossible that one B vitamin could influence so many different parts of us and so many different aspects of ill health and poisoning that may affect us, and yet the following case histories from medical journals and other sources reveal a wide variety of effects of vitamin B_6 on human health. They lead us to think that doctors generally are not doing nearly enough with vitamin B_6 and other vitamins and minerals in treating the numerous disorders that plague us.

Nutrition Reviews for September, 1966 gives us some evidence that vitamin B_6 is essential for the normal functioning of the pituitary gland. This is an important endocrine gland located at the base of the brain. Hormones from this gland regulate growth and apparently control the secretions of other endocrine glands, such as the thyroid and adrenals.

The authors point out that lack of pyridoxine is likely to produce slow growth in children. It is also true, say these authors, that the normal pituitary gland contains a rather high content of vitamin B_6, suggesting that it is, indeed, important for the function of this mastergland of the body.

Homocysteinuria is an inherited disorder in which mental retardation may develop, and in which abnormal amounts of a certain compound are excreted in the urine, because of the absence of a certain enzyme activity.

The Lancet for June 24, 1967 reported on reversal of abnormalities in three patients with this disease, plus experience with two more patients in whom most of the distressing symptoms were reversed when very large doses of pyridoxine were given. One 10-year-old boy was given 500 milligrams of pyridoxine daily by mouth. A four-year-old girl, given 300 milligrams of the B vitamin daily, showed reversal of most abnormal symptoms until she got an attack of chickenpox which set back her recovery. Later, when she was given 500 milligrams of the B vitamin daily, she showed great improvement.

Notice that in all cases where pyridoxine has been given in large amounts, no mention is made of unpleasant or dangerous side effects. There are none.

Hydrazine is a volatile chemical which is widely used in industry as a corrosion inhibitor and in the military as a rocket propellant. In laboratory animals, reports the *New England Journal of Medicine*, April 22, 1976, it produces convulsions, circulatory collapse, lung edema, hypoglycemia, vomiting, intestitial nephritis and liver damage. Chronic exposure to hydrazine can produce in human beings pneumonia, liver damage, nephritis and other kidney damage. There may also be seizures or convulsions.

"Pyridoxine is an effective antidote against hydrazine-induced seizures in rats, but has rarely been reported as an antidote for human hydrazine poisoning," says the *Journal*.

They report on a man brought to the Massachusetts General Hospital after an accident in an industrial procedure involving hydrazine. Fourteen hours later he went into a coma and remained comatose for 60 hours.

The doctors decided to use pyridoxine. They injected 600 milligrams intramuscularly slowly in a continuous infusion over three hours. One hour later he opened his eyes and shortly thereafter his mental capacity returned to normal. He recalled everything that had happened to him at the accident site. Careful investigation revealed no brain damage. Several other similar cases are reported in the same article.

Doesn't it seem possible that toxicity from other chemicals might also be treated with this harmless B vitamin? Since it is harmless in even very large doses, is there any reason not to try it, especially when the damage is being done to nerve and brain tissues?

In 1960, Dr. Michael G. Wohl of the Hahnemann Medical College reported in *Proceedings of the Society for Experi-*

mental Biology and Medicine that pyridoxine is lacking in the person suffering from hyperthyroidism, that is, a thyroid gland that is too active.

Handbook of Vitamins and Hormones by Roman J. Kutsky tells us that hyperthyroid individuals are likely to be short on the entire B complex of vitamins. This suggests that if you are having thyroid problems of any nature it might be wise to be sure you are getting enough of all the B vitamins, just to be sure that any deficiency will be taken care of.

Chloramphenicol (chloromycetin) is an antibiotic which is capable of causing such extremely serious side effects that it is not often used except in those diseases where no other drug is effective.

Yet doctors in 1967 reported in the *American Journal of Diseases of Children* that very high doses of pyridoxine and vitamin B_{12} prevented the optic nerve condition that had bothered their patient when previous doses of the antibiotic were given. The authors of the article suggest that, when this very dangerous drug must be given, very large doses of these two B vitamins should always accompany it. It seems possible to us that other harmful drugs might also turn out to be far less of a risk if large doses of these vitamins were given.

Annals of Internal Medicine, volume 59, page 724, 1963, reported on a man who had no symptoms of pyridoxine deficiency. But he was suffering from mild anemia and "severe" neuropathy. That is, many kinds of severe nerve problems. He was given large doses of pyridoxine and both the anemia and the nerve problems cleared up.

The B complex of vitamins, given during the first three months of pregnancy, may have a lot to do with preventing birth defects such as cleft palate, according to researchers at St. Barnabas Medical Center in Newark, N. J. and reported in the *Journal of the American Medical Association* for July 27, 1963.

They studied 576 pregnant women. A group of 418 of

these were given vitamin therapy and 158 had none. Of the women who got no vitamin B supplements during pregnancy, 7.9 percent gave birth to children with deformities, while birth defects occurred in the babies of only 3.8 percent of the women who got the B vitamins.

Some of the women in both groups had a family history of birth defects. But, regardless of this, the B vitamins brought about a lower incidence of defects. A tablet consisting of the complete B complex was given, along with 10 milligrams of pyridoxine and 5 milligrams of folic acid, another B vitamin.

We all know the effects of sugar and sticky sweets on teeth. We know, too, that lack of minerals like calcium can make the teeth less able to resist the decay caused by sticky sweets. But did you know that the B vitamin pyridoxine has a very helpful effect in preventing tooth decay? *The American Journal of Clinical Nutrition* (June, 1962) presented the experience of a group of 540 pregnant women, some of whom were given pyridoxine supplements.

Records of the DMF (decayed, missing, filled) teeth of all the women were available. They were checked again after delivery of the babies. The patients who had the pyridoxine supplements showed, on the average, a smaller increase in decayed, missing and filled teeth than the comparison group, all of whom got no extra pyridoxine in their diets.

Many older folks suffer from lack of hydrochloric acid in the stomach. Without enough of this digestive juice food is not digested normally and the patient suffers agonies of indigestion or "chronic gastritis" as the doctors call it.

A Soviet doctor reported in 1965 that giving pyridoxine orally increased the production of this essential digestive juice and put an end to the distress in 18 of 30 patients complaining of it. He also suggested that people with stomach ulcers should probably not use large doses of pyridoxine since it may increase their stomach acidity, as well.

In 1964 Dr. Carroll M. Leevy of the Seton Hall College of Medicine told a session of the 45th annual meeting of the American College of Physicians that he had studied 172 alcoholics with and without liver disease or symptoms of vitamin deficiency and found that lack of certain B vitamins—chiefly folic acid, vitamin B_{12} and pyridoxine—accentuated the destructive effects of alcohol on the liver.

The liver has a great capacity to recover and regenerate healthy cells when it is damaged. But it must have enough of the important vitamins for this regenerative process to take place. If they are not present, there is an upward spiral of greater and greater liver damage. The drinker's diet usually consists of nothing much but alcohol, with sandwiches and snacks. There is almost no vitamin B content in such a diet. The liver damaged by alcohol finally becomes so damaged that it cannot utilize any vitamins it needs, even if they are supplied in ample quantity.

Said Dr. Leevy, "alcoholics can be suffering from severe vitamin deficiences without showing any of the easily recognizable signs of deficiency—such as nerve damage, anemia and skin disorders."

Even giving thiamine, the B vitamin lack of which is most usually associated with an alcoholic's problems, does not solve the problem. Deficiency in other B vitamins (pyridoxine for instance) may be so severe that the liver is too damaged to make use of the thiamine (B_1).

A peculiar thing about pyridoxine that turned up in *Nutrition Reviews* for February, 1973 shows that animals which are deficient in this B vitamin are more likely to have trouble clearing from their blood the seasoning agent MSG (monosodium glutamate). This is the seasoning agent used extensively in Chinese food which causes some people to have uncomfortable and frightening nervous symptoms. MSG was also found to be quite dangerous in the early days of life for infant animals.

So, if you are a devotee of Chinese food and want to eat it without an unpleasant reaction to the MSG it contains, you might try fortifying yourself with a dose of pyridoxine before you start out for the restaurant.

As long ago as 1963 the *American Journal of Clinical Nutrition* reported that vitamin B₆ is important in helping the body deal with fatty foods. Fats, including the pesty cholesterol, decreased in the blood when large doses of pyridoxine were given. In the welter of commercials for low-cholesterol foods, has anyone ever announced that simply by taking a bit more of a harmless B vitamin you can overcome any tendency to high blood levels of cholesterol?

A report in the *Annals of the Society for Experimental Biology and Medicine* in August, 1961 revealed that rats which are placed on a diet in which there is little or no pyridoxine have very high levels of cholesterol in their blood. The aorta, the blood vessel close to the heart which is afflicted in heart attacks, showed gross deposits of fatty substances when pyridoxine was removed from the animals' diets. This suggests certainly that the fears of modern-day Americans where cholesterol is concerned might easily be alleviated by just getting enough pyridoxine every day.

In 1965 a New York City researcher, Dr. Edward H. Mandel, reported that pyridoxine has anti-coagulant activity—that is, it can prevent the abnormal and unwanted clotting of blood, as in circulatory disorders. Many strokes and heart attacks are apparently caused by blood that coagulates abnormally and forms blood clots which then migrate to heart, lungs or brain, causing stoppages in the flow of blood which brings about the damage in cases of heart attacks or strokes.

Three vitamins are involved in the body's production of antibodies, those substances which protect us from infections of all kinds. These three are pyridoxine, pantothenic acid and vitamin C, according to Dr. A. E. Axelrod, professor of biochemistry at the University of Pittsburgh School of Medicine. Without these three powerful substances rats show a decreasing amount of antibodies—those compounds which would protect them from diphtheria and flu viruses.

The way in which pyridoxine creates its effects has to do with its role in producing RNA and DNA, those two substances which exist in every cell and which are essential for the body to create protein out of amino acids in food. The antibodies are made of protein and must be constructed from the protein in our diets.

The September, 1962 issue of the *American Journal of Clinical Nutrition* printed the results of an experiment to test the ability of pyridoxine to protect against infections. It was quite a strenuous test, we think.

Six men were fed a diet from which all pyridoxine had been removed, and all other known nutrients retained. Then two of them received a drug that is known to deplete the body of pyridoxine. So, to all intents and purposes, there was no pyridoxine in the bodies of these two men. Two men served as controls and were given pyridoxine.

Then all of them were injected with tetanus and typhoid shots. The men who had been given pyridoxine remained well throughout. The men who had been deliberately made deficient in pyridoxine all became ill. Ample proof that this one vitamin alone protects against infectious diseases.

Two 1966 reports from the Soviet Union show that vitamin B_6 is effective in the treatment of chronic hepatitis and cirrhosis of the liver. The vitamin was given along with vitamin B_{12} in doses of 700 to 1,000 milligrams for 15-20 days. The liver conditions began to improve only after the B vitamins were given.

Herpes gestationis is a blistery skin eruption that sometimes occurs in pregnancy. *Archives of Dermatology* for June, 1965 tells the story of a case of this unpleasant condition which developed in the fourth week of pregnancy. The patient did not respond to hormone drugs. But when 10 milligrams of pyridoxine were given daily there was a "dramatic" remission. And the B vitamin was given only until the 25th week of pregnancy, then discontinued. The skin disorder did not return.

For the life of us we cannot conceive of why this mild, harmless dose of this helpful vitamin was discontinued, when it was very obvious that the woman was deficient in this B vitamin. Why not just go on taking it for life merely to guard against any other kind of disorder that might appear due to lack of pyridoxine in meals or due to a much higher requirement than average?

CHAPTER 2

Vitamin B$_6$
"The Sleeping Giant"

EXECUTIVE HEALTH for November, 1975 calls pyridoxine "the sleeping giant of nutrition." Most nutrition experts agree that this vitamin has had not nearly the extensive research that other vitamins have had. It was not until 1953 that its absolute need for life and health was proven, thus establishing it as a vitamin.

All animals require this vitamin. It is essential for the body's processing of all proteins, carbohydrates and fats, which makes it the cornerstone of a good digestive system. Of special importance these days is its function in dealing with proteins and fats. It also takes part in enzyme systems which produce neural hormones—those body substances that regulate and activate our nerves. It is also essential for directing the pathways of unsaturated fats in our bodies, regulating bile acids which are concerned with digesting fats, forming certain kinds of red blood cells and promoting growth in children.

According to Roman J. Kutsky, deficiency diseases which appear when pyridoxine is lacking are hardening of the arteries (in monkeys) and acrodynia in rats. This is a disorder involving extreme irritability alternating with periods of apathy, lack of appetite, pink itching feet, profuse sweating, rapid heartbeat, high blood pressure and often flaking skin on feet.

In human beings, says Kutsky, deficiency in pyridoxine can produce: convulsions, dermatitis, irritability, nervous disorders and lymphopenia (reduction in the amount of lymph).

Thirty to thirty-four percent of all the pyridoxine in our food can be lost in cooking, especially when the water in which food was cooked is thrown away. Any drug or condition which causes diuresis (excessive urination) brings about loss of pyridoxine. Any disease of the digestive and intestinal tract brings about loss of pyridoxine. Irradiation, too, causes us to lose this extremely valuable B vitamin.

Some symptoms we may be able to notice ourselves which indicate lack of pyridoxine are: skin troubles, anemia and nerve disorders including convulsions. Doctors test us for pyridoxine deficiency by looking for a certain substance (xanthurenic acid) in the urine.

Can you get too much pyridoxine? Well, Kutsky states that there is "limited toxicity." Human beings have shown disturbing symptoms when they were getting 3 grams per kilogram of weight. This means that a 150-pound man would have to take 225 *grams* of pyridoxine before he would show signs of getting too much. Since pyridoxine is measured out in pills consisting of milligrams, which are thousandths of a gram, it is easy to see that it would be almost impossible for anyone to show signs of toxicity from taking even very large doses of this water-soluble vitamin.

In laboratory animals where researchers can produce absolute deficiency in the vitamin by carefully designed diets they can produce many symptoms which appear to be closely related to many conditions of ill health that are troubling present-day Americans.

Animals made deficient in pyridoxine excrete more urea and show increased urea in their blood. (Increased urea is a symptom of gout in human beings.) Animals made deficient in pyridoxine excrete more oxalate. (Oxalate is the basis of kidney stones in human beings, indicating that something has gone wrong to produce excretion of much more than is normal of this compound.)

Animals made deficient in pyridoxine have too little insulin. (Insulin is lacking in human diabetics.) Animals made deficient in pyridoxine show demyelinization of nerves. This is the destruction of the myelin sheaths of the nerves. Polio and multiple sclerosis are two human diseases in which the myelin sheaths of the nerves are being destroyed. Animals made deficient in pyridoxine have convulsions. Human babies have convulsions when they are not getting as much pyridoxine as they need, and many have far larger needs than the "average" person needs.

How is pyridoxine related to the other vitamins? It works with pantothenic acid (another B vitamin). A deficiency in both results in lowered concentrations of an essential body enzyme. A deficiency in both vitamin B_{12} and pyridoxine results in reduced absorption and storage of vitamin B_{12}. Vitamin E and pyridoxine work together to control the body's use of the unsaturated fats.

When pyridoxine is deficient, more vitamin C is excreted. The conversion of vitamin C to oxalates is increased when not enough pyridoxine is present. People who are worried about kidney stones being formed when too much vitamin C is taken should take pyridoxine to prevent the formation of these oxalate stones. Plenty of vitamin C, on the other hand, helps to alleviate some of the deficiency symptoms of pyridoxine. The two vitamins work together in handling one of the amino acids, tyrosine.

Pyridoxine helps in the process of breaking down another amino acid tryptophan into niacin (vitamin B_3). An overdose of thiamine (vitamin B_1) can bring about deficiency in pyridoxine. Vitamin B_2 (riboflavin) and biotin (another B vitamin) work along with pyridoxine in the body. All these complex interrelationships underline the necessity *for always taking the B vitamins as a group*. If you want to take larger doses of one or another, always be sure you are taking, in addition, at least some of the entire B complex of vitamins, to avoid any related deficiency in one or another.

Kutsky lists 14 body hormones which are closely involved with pyridoxine. Among them are insulin, several hormones of the adrenal glands (which protect us from stress) and a number of sex hormones.

To get back to *Executive Health*, we find a number of references to ways in which all these essential activities of pyridoxine show up in various body functions, especially when they are not working normally. For example, some women and girls suffer outbreaks of acne just before their menstrual periods. In a recent experiment 72 percent of those taking 50 milligrams of pyridoxine daily for one week before and during their periods had no further problems with acne.

Large amounts of fat in the diets of rhesus monkeys call for increased amounts of pyridoxine. It takes five milligrams of pyridoxine a day to protect them from cholesterol deposits caused by deficiency in this B vitamin. Translating this into human terms, this means that an adult man would need at least 25 milligrams of pyridoxine daily if he is eating a diet high in fat and cholesterol, as most Americans are.

Some children suffer from breath-holding spells. In apparent rage, they can hold their breath until their faces turn blue from lack of oxygen. Concerned parents try many kinds of psychological ploys to avoid these frightening incidents. *Executive Health* tells us that plenty of pyridoxine in the child's diet prevents these incidents.

One pediatrician has reported that for 10 years he has been treating breath-holding spells with 40 milligrams of pyridoxine a day for children up to two years old, 40 milligrams twice a day for older children, for a period of one month. He has gotten, he said, excellent results. He reported in a study printed in a professional journal on child neurology that he believes there may be a definite metabolic disorder in children who have these breath-holding spells. This disorder seems to arise from deficiency in pyridoxine. Giving the vitamin stops the breath-holding tendency because it corrects the metabolic disorder.

One kind of anemia which, for some reason, occurs almost exclusively in men, can be prevented and treated with pyridoxine. The B vitamin can relieve the neuritic pain produced by some drugs. Orthomolecular psychiatrists are using pyridoxine successfully in addition to other B vitamins to treat mentally ill patients. It is also being used to treat arthritis.

Beriberi is caused by deficiency in the B vitamin thiamine. Pellagra is caused by deficiency in the B vitamin niacin. But way back in the 1930's when pellagra was still plaguing hundreds of thousands of people in our South, physicians found that the disease often returned after it had been treated with niacin. They then gave pyridoxine and the symptoms disappeared within 24 hours. "One man," says the magazine, "unable to walk more than a few steps before the injection, walked two miles the day afterward." This is another indication of the complex interrelationships among B vitamins.

According to official statements of the National Academy of Sciences, the average adult needs only 1½ to 2 milligrams of pyridoxine daily. Yet in a study of mentally ill children, the need for the vitamin was found to vary all the way from five milligrams a day to 400 milligrams!

According to some reports as many as 34 percent of all women who use The Pill (the oral contraceptive) suffer from depression which may be mild to moderate, also irritability, as well as swings from emotional highs to lows, lethargy and fatigue. Some may develop paranoid tendencies, that is, they imagine that they are being unjustly persecuted. As many as 75 percent of such women have been markedly improved when pyridoxine was added to their supplements—50 milligrams a day. Pyridoxine also seems to be effective in stopping lactation in women who do not breast-feed their babies. Up to now doctors have used the female hormone, estrogen, to accomplish this. The hormone has produced some undesirable side effects such as rebound filling of the breasts and increased susceptibility to strokes caused by abnormal clotting of the blood.

A report in the *British Journal of Obstetrics and Gynecology*, Volume 80; page 718, 1973 told of 254 women in which pyridoxine relieved breast engorgement and led to complete and normal suppression of milk formation within one week for all of the women. There were no undesirable side effects.

To sum up, said *Executive Health*, "Good nutrition should begin with the unborn child and be continued from infancy throughout life if crippling and deadly diseases are to be prevented. And it would seem that it must include a goodly supply of vitamin B_6 which, although bountiful in nature, has been largely removed from our foods by overprocessing and overcooking.

A severe form of anemia may develop in dogs and swine which are being fed diets deficient in vitamin B_6, reports the Vitamin Information Bureau, Inc. Red blood cells are pale, small and tend to vary greatly in size and shape. Blood iron levels are high, iron storage in bone marrow and liver is increased, and siderocytes (red cells with iron deposits) are seen. Vitamin B_6 therapy corrects the problem.

Recently, an anemia with similar blood picture, clinical course and response to vitamin B_6 therapy has been found in man, the bureau says. Of 72 patients tabulated by Hines and Harris, nine were children. The condition responds to about 25 milligrams of pyridoxine per day, and most patients apparently require a maintenance dose of vitamin B_6 to keep the anemia under control. However, the bureau states, the blood picture is not completely restored to normal even with B_6 therapy.

The condition, called pyridoxine-dependent anemia, runs in families and, therefore, may be of genetic origin. Investigators in Manchester, England studied a large family in which five affected members, all middle-aged men, were found. Since no women were found with the disorder in the family, investigators speculated that the condition, like hemophilia, may be an X-linked recessive trait. Whatever the mode of inheritance, the bureau continues, the hereditary factor in some way interferes with B_6 utilization or greatly increases its requirements.

There is also a B_6-responsive anemia that has been seen in tuberculosis patients treated with the standard anti-TB drug, isoniazid (INH), the bureau reports. "The drug is a chemical antagonist of B_6 and itself produces pyridoxine deficiency, accompanied by nervous system effects. Anemia, however, is a very rare complication, since only six or seven cases have been reported. Treatment with B_6 promptly corrected the anemia without need to discontinue INH and other anti-TB drugs," the bureau says.

The Vitamin Information Bureau also reports that a vitamin B_6 deficiency in some fashion produces brain dysfunction which is manifested as abnormal electroencephalographic (EEG) tracings and outright convulsions. This has led many investigators to look for possible abnormalities in B6 metabolism in certain kinds of epilepsy of unknown origin.

At the 9th International Congress of Pediatrics in Montreal, Canada, in 1959, W. A. Cochrane reported on five patients with "infantile spasms" described as lightning fits, the bureau says. The infants had positive tryptophan (amino acid) load test, indicating some abnormality in pyridoxine metabolism. They received supplemental B_6 therapy, which Cochrane felt improved their mental status and lessened convulsions.

Since then Bengt Hagbergand in Uppsala, Sweden and B. D. Bower and associates in Birmingham, England have studied the relation between forms of childhood epilepsy and B_6 metabolism, apparently with little results.

"Extensive work-up on many children with infantile spasms did not show that their patients had B_6 deficiency; their diet seemed adequate and blood levels of B_6 were usually normal," the bureau reports. "Nor was there much to indicate that the children as a group were B_6-dependent. B_6 treatment generally did not produce clinical improvement (five of 56 cases in the Swedish study benefited)."

However, the bureau continues, the investigators feel that the available data suggest that some of the patients with infantile spasms are afflicted with defective utilization of B_6. The Birmingham group found similar signs in an unexpectedly large number of controls with non-epileptic diseases of the central nervous system (mental retardation, spastic paraplegia; cerebral palsy, etc.)

CHAPTER 3

Are We Getting Enough Vitamin B6?

A REPORT FROM the National Vitamin Foundation asks "Are We Consuming Enough Vitamin B6?" This is a report on an address by Dr. W. H. Sebrell, Jr. of the Institute of Nutrition Sciences, Columbia University, New York.

Said Dr. Sebrell, "In view of the possibility that large numbers of people in this country may be eating diets which furnish less than desirable amounts of vitamin B6, there is a particularly urgent need for acquiring new knowledge about vitamin B6 as rapidly as possible to determine both the requirement and the intake of the vitamin. Some investigators believe that a surprisingly high percentage of Americans are not getting enough of this vital nutrient in their meals."

Typical home and restaurant meals analyzed in laboratory tests conducted at the Massachusetts Institute of Technology were found to contain much less vitamin B6 than expected, indicating significant losses of the vitamin during the processing and preparation of food.

"Viewing the situation as a whole, there is a strong case for increasing the B6 in the food supply," says Dr. Henry Borsook of the California Institute of Technology. He pointed out that the high intake of protein in most American meals increases the need for pyridoxine, that pregnant women, el-

22

derly persons and those on weight reducing diets may not be getting enough of the vitamin. He believes, he said, that pyridoxine should be added to all flour and bread, as three other B vitamins are added now.

"If enrichment with thiamine and riboflavin is called for," said Dr. Borsook, "then the call is even greater for enrichment with B_6." The third B vitamin generally added to flour and bread is B_3 (niacin).

B_6 is called the "amino acid metabolism vitamin" because of its prominence in enzyme systems involved in the use of amino acids, or building blocks of protein, in the human body. Its basic function is to help in the efficient use of protein and fat, to build and rebuild vital tissue and supply needed energy.

We know that pyridoxine is essential for manufacturing human hemoglobin thus preventing anemia. Anemic patients who would not respond to any other treatment have been cured when pyridoxine was given. Vitamin B_6 is also essential for the normal function of the nervous system. In infants the most striking sign of lack of this vitamin is convulsions. Deficiency at any age causes tension, irritability and even severe mental illness. (Sound like anybody you know?)

"Abnormal B_6 metabolism affects the central nervous system and alters brain function," says Dr. David Baird Coursin of Lancaster, Pa. "In infants with an inborn error of metabolism, or with an acquired defect, large doses of the vitamin are necessary to prevent not only abnormalities of chemical energetics but also structural changes that become irreversible. . . . It is quite conceivable that such changes may produce a persistent tendency to convulsive seizures as well as result in permanent retardation."

Large doses of vitamin B_6 have been found to be effective in the treatment of liver conditions, especially in alcoholics whose diets are generally very deficient in many nutrients.

Those with various skin ailments have also benefited from

the vitamin, as well as individuals in special situations of risk like radiation exposure, heart failure and those given various drugs for the treatment of tuberculosis.

Another possible role of great significance for the vitamin, said Dr. Sebrell, is the formation of antibodies which help to protect us from infectious diseases. "Since vitamin B_6 is so deeply involved in protein metabolism," he said, "it would not be surprising to find that it has an important function in the immunological processes of the body. This is a field which calls for careful study in the evaluation of our need for vitamin B_6."

Many studies have shown that laboratory animals made deficient in vitamin B_6, then injected with diphtheria, typhoid, tetanus or flu, produce not only fewer antibodies to combat the invading disease, but also weaker ones. Studies with human beings have shown the same thing to be true. Interestingly, in these men there was an even greater reduction in the defenses of the body when another B vitamin, pantothenic acid, was also deficient.

At the April, 1974 meeting of the Federation of Societies for Experimental Biology, papers were presented on some new aspects of vitamins and minerals.

Six scientists reported on a study of the vitamin B_6 status of American men. They studied 617 men aged 18 to 90—all clinically healthy, educated men who had plenty of money to buy nourishing food and supposedly enough good nutritional sense to know which foods are nourishing. About one-third of these men were taking vitamin B_6 supplements— anywhere from 0.1 to 105 milligrams of this B vitamin every day.

The average amount of the vitamin found in the blood of men who were *not* taking supplements was below a level of 10 which is the lowest "acceptable" limit. Seven percent of these showed blood that was definitely deficient in pyridoxine. If the supplement contained less than 2 milligrams daily, the amount in the blood was still below desirable levels.

In another study, three scientists from Florida State University asked students about their diets and calculated the amounts of vitamin B_6 such diets contain. *They found that three-fourths of the students were actually getting in their food less vitamin B_6 than the Recommended Dietary Allowances advise.* There seems to be no relation between the amount of the vitamin eaten and the amount of usable pyridoxine in the blood, which seemed to indicate, say these researchers, that there is a wide variation in individual requirements for this B vitamin.

Years ago this vitamin was destroyed in the preparation of certain commercially available baby formulas. A number of babies died in convulsions before anyone discovered that the trouble was the pyridoxine-deficient formulas. Others suffered from convulsions but managed to live. Other babies who had the same formulas suffered no harm. This was an early indication that the individual requirements for this vitamin vary widely. If you happen to be one of those people whose requirement is very high, you may come to some serious trouble if you do not supply your body with enough pyridoxine.

In the years since 1974 we have seen nothing to indicate that this situation in regard to pyridoxine deficiency has changed. It's just that nobody has done any more surveys.

CHAPTER 4

A Startling New Theory on the Cause of Hardening of the Arteries

TWO NEUROPHYSIOLOGISTS at the Massachusetts Institute of Technology have written an article entitled "Beyond Cholesterol", in which they challenge the present theory that cholesterol in our meals is the basic cause of hardening of the arteries and heart attacks. And what is even more scandalous, they published their article in a layman's magazine, *Atlantic*, rather than a scientific journal. They are writing a book on their theory, which will also be addressed to plain non-scientists.

Their actions have outraged a number of defenders of the cholesterol theory who pronounce the new theory not only worthless but nonsensical. And yet, somehow, we have a feeling that the new theory is bound to be proven at least partly valid. Undoubtedly, what Edward R. Gruberg and Stephen A. Raymond say in their fine *Atlantic* article sounds very reasonable to us. And it is easy to understand how professional scientists and nutritionists who have made their living for the past 10 years promoting the cholesterol theory will be forced to declare the new theory suspect.

It hinges on a B vitamin. That alone is enough to curl the hair and bare the teeth of your average defender of fake eggs and diets low in cholesterol. The vitamin is pyridoxine. The theory goes like this, greatly over-simplified. The amino acid (form of protein) called methionine is essential for human health and must be obtained from food. It is most abundant in foods of animal origin—meat, poultry, fish, dairy products and eggs. But these foods do not contain as much pyridoxine as do foods of vegetable origin.

It seems that methionine breaks down in the body into several substances, one of which is called homocysteine. This breakdown product can become very troublesome unless there is enough pyridoxine on hand to detoxify it and get it carried away harmlessly in the urine. Since diets high in animal protein don't contain a great deal of pyridoxine and since this vitamin is readily destroyed when any food is cooked, it appears likely that many of us modern Americans, eating lots of animal products, may be short on pyridoxine.

As a result, we may be suffering from a residue of homocysteine in our blood and tissues. How does this affect us? A number of years ago, two Irish children who were mentally deficient were found to have very high levels of homocysteine in their urine. The substance was being excreted without being normally processed in the body. The doctors who found this disorder duly reported it and eventually other children were found with this same problem which was apparently inherited.

Autopsies on a number of these children (from seven to thirteen years of age) revealed that all were suffering from "extensive" hardening of the arteries and blood clots. These are conditions which are usually associated with older people, as well as those with various diseases like diabetes, high blood pressure and so on. The children had none of these diseases. So their doctors could only assume that it was the overload of homocysteine in their little bodies which produced the artery hardening. They named the disease *homocysteinuria*, indicating that its most significant symptom was large amounts of this breakdown product in their urine.

In 1969 Dr. Kilmer McCully, professor of pathology at Harvard Medical School, came to the conclusion that the disease from which these children suffered was only "the tip of the iceberg." He reasoned that pyridoxine is essential for processing homocysteine in the body and if enough of this B vitamin is not present, something will go wrong with the process. Hardening of the arteries may be the result in older folks as well as in children.

He found that in 1948 University of California researchers had fed monkeys a diet deficient in pyridoxine and produced hardening of the arteries. Deficiencies in other B vitamins did not produce this result. Nobody paid much attention to this finding, but Dr. McCully went on with his research. He theorized that if not enough pyridoxine is present in human blood, the homocysteine will not be disposed of correctly and this harmful substance will accumulate in the blood.

Cholesterol is a normal component of human blood. *But homocysteine is not.* So it accumulates and causes hardening of the arteries. Dr. McCully thought he might be able to show that animals with large amounts of homocysteine in their blood will get hardening of the arteries. And human beings and animals who do not have enough vitamin B_6 may show large amounts of homocysteine in their blood. People who are known to have hardening of the arteries should also be proven to be deficient in pyridoxine. And they should have too much homocysteine in their blood.

All of these suppositions proved to be true. In rabbits and in baboons homocysteine was shown to produce hardening of the arteries. "It is much more potent than cholesterol," say our authors, "even when cholesterol is given in such huge doses that it becomes a major dietary nutrient."

Then a study on human beings showed that when they were on a diet devoid of pyridoxine, they began to excrete homocysteine. Work done here and in Russia also showed that coronary patients have much lower blood levels of pyridoxine than healthy people—about one quarter as much. Finally, experiments in Australia have shown that coronary patients are much more likely to have homocysteine in their blood than are people who are relatively free of hardening of the arteries.

"Vitamin B_6 is the key to the clearing of homocysteine from the blood," say Gruberg and Raymond. Looking at a

---

Methionine and Pyridoxine in 100 Grams of Some Foods

Food	Methionine Milligrams	Pyridoxine Milligrams
Eggs	360	0.110
Milk, whole	93	0.40
Liver	530	0.65 to 0.84
Beef, raw	515	0.33
Fish	610	0.17
Wheat germ	330	1.15
Soybean meal	760	0.724
Brown rice	205	0.550
Potatoes, raw	50	0.250
Whole oats	230	0.14
Barley	190	0.22
Brewers yeast	1,395	2.50
Whole corn	250	0.25
Peanut flour and butter	550 (flour)	0.330 (Butter)
Dried peas and beans, raw	460	0.580

The listing of methionine comes from a list of essential amino acids in foods, listed in decreasing order of their biologic (nutritional) value. The pyridoxine figures are from U.S.D.A. *Home Economics Research Report No. 36.*

---

list of foods that contain this vitamin and then noting that the official recommendation is only two milligrams a day, it seems impossible that so many Americans would be short on this vitamin. But keep in mind that the important thing here is the ratio between the methionine in the diet and the pyridoxine. The more methionine you eat, the more pyridoxine you need to process it correctly.

A serving of beef contains 970 milligrams of methionine and only half a milligram of pyridoxine. Cheese contains 653 milligrams of methionine and only 7/100 milligram of pyridoxine. Chicken contains 537 milligrams of methionine and only ½ milligram of pyridoxine. Peanut butter contains 256 milligrams of methionine and ⅓ milligram of pyridoxine. Yogurt contains 102 milligrams of methionine and 3/100 milligram of pyridoxine.

Now don't get the idea that you should immediately stop eating any foods that contain methionine. It comes along with protein wherever protein appears in food. Meat, eggs, poultry and dairy products contain more methionine than most vegetarian foods. This is one reason why they are more valuable nutritionally than most vegetarian foods—because methionine is absolutely essential for good health and it does not occur in very large amounts in those vegetarian foods which have low protein content like fruits, carrots, lettuce, potatoes, tomatoes and so on. The vegetarian foods are, relatively speaking, far richer in pyridoxine than the foods of animal origin.

So the lesson to be learned is to eat plenty of those good foods which contain methionine and also plenty of those foods which contain lots of pyridoxine. In this way, you get a balance which will (according to this new theory) maintain good health without risk of hardening of the arteries. Which foods, then, should be avoided? Only those foods *which make up half the diet of many Americans*—the refined carbohydrates. Practically all the pyridoxine has been removed from such foods.

White bread contains only 4/100 of a milligram of pyridoxine. Sugar, of course, contains not a bit of pyridoxine, since all the B vitamins have been removed from sugar. Several other B vitamins are returned to bread flour, BUT NOT PYRIDOXINE. So you can see that a daily sandwich of meat and white bread with no fruit, no vegetables, plus a dessert of cake or pie would contain considerable amounts of methionine and practically no pyridoxine to guarantee normal breakdown of the methionine in the digestive tract and blood.

Let's say such a lunch is followed by a dinner of meat or poultry, plus potatoes and lots more white bread, plus another sugary dessert. Once again, you would have lots of methionine and practically no pyridoxine to protect you from the build-up of the abnormal homocysteine which is a breakdown product of methionine.

Remember, too, that whatever pyridoxine does exist in meat and bread is mostly destroyed when they are cooked. This suggests that raw fruits and vegetables are an absolute essential for a healthful diet. Salads in some form should accompany every meal you eat. Fresh, raw fruit should accompany every meal you eat.

Vitamin B_6 is a water soluble vitamin. It is present in every all-in-one vitamin preparation in varying amounts. The amount you need is an entirely individual matter which no one can predict. A woman taking The Pill needs far larger amounts of this vitamin than the rest of us. The *Atlantic* authors tell us that a recent investigation of 46,000 English women included 23,000 taking The Pill and 23,000 who were not taking The Pill. The death rate in the still relatively young women who had taken The Pill continuously for five years or more *was ten times that* of those who had never taken The Pill. According to the new theory, lack of pyridoxine could be the major factor in this tragic finding.

Other drugs which destroy pyridoxine in the body are the hydralazine family of drugs, given to control high blood pressure. Since high blood pressure is one accompanying symptom of hardening of the arteries, it seems possible, does it not, that these drugs may be making matters worse by destroying the very vitamin that might be preventing the original condition for which the drugs are prescribed! The drug penicillamine also destroys pyridoxine. This drug is given to treat Wilson's Disease. It is also advocated for use in arthritis, scleroderma and schizophrenia. L-dopa, which is given for Parkinson's Disease, is also destructive of vitamin B_6.

A large number of our fellow citizens are taking such drugs as these. Are these the same people who suffer from artery hardening? Who knows? Until and unless the new theory on pyridoxine is investigated there is no way to know. We do know that needs for pyridoxine vary widely.

Should you take additional vitamin B_6 in an effort to avoid hardening of the arteries? Of course, you should. And you should, in addition, try to maintain the balance in your meals that is suggested above. Sure, eat plenty of high protein foods, both animal and vegetable. You need this high quality protein and you need all the vitamins and minerals these foods contain. But be certain to balance this kind of diet with plenty of fruits and vegetables, preferably raw, since cooking is very destructive of pyridoxine. The only foods you should make a determined effort to avoid in order to test this new theory are the refined carbohydrates—white sugar and white flour in any form or any food.

In addition, don't decide, on the basis of the new theory, that you can ignore all the other aspects of diet and way of life that have been shown to be involved in the production of poor circulatory health. Don't smoke. Don't drink. Cut down on all drugs such as coffee, strong tea, soft drinks, sugar and over-the-counter drugs. Get plenty of exercise, every day of your life—purposeful, vigorous exercise.

As we were completing this book, the Food and Nutrition Board of the National Research Council in Washington, D.C., announced that "it had found no reason for the average healthy American to restrict consumption of cholesterol," reported the *New York Times*, May 28, 1980. The board, a division of the National Academy of Sciences, added that fat intake should not be reduced "except as necessary to achieve and maintain a normal body weight."

The board did suggest that overweight Americans should reduce dietary fat, exercise more and confine their alcohol consumption to at or below the equivalent of three mixed drinks a day. Fat, which is a source of more than twice as many calories as the equivalent amount of protein or carbohydrate, and alcohol are concentrated sources of nutritionally empty calories, the board suggested.

In another move, the board urged Americans to reduce their salt intake to between three and eight grams a day, as compared with the 10 grams that most people consume.

The cholesterol and fat recommendations understandably drew immediate flack from some food companies and health associations, who have been thriving for years with foods and statements which have implicated cholesterol as the main cause of heart disease and circulatory problems. It will not be easy for them to back-track so swiftly, especially since millions of dollars in food sales, advertising budgets, etc., are at stake.

CHAPTER 5

Pyridoxine May Help to Prevent Bladder Cancer

CANCER OF the urinary bladder appears to be an increasing threat as the toxins in our environment accumulate at a frightening pace and less and less is known about their potential for causing cancer. The body has defense mechanisms for disposing of poisons. It eliminates them as rapidly as possible. One method is to excrete them in urine. So it seems possible that many of the poisons to which we are exposed daily find their way to the kidney, then to the bladder by way of the ureter, which is the connecting tube between these two organs.

It might surprise you to hear that some substances suspected of causing bladder cancer are things some of us use every day, some of us use at every meal. The June 23, 1973 issue of the *Canadian Medical Journal* contained an article on the subject by Balfour M. Mount of the Department of Urology at the Royal Victoria Hospital and the Department of Surgery at McGill University in Montreal.

Dr. Mount tells us the earliest discovery of a relationship between environmental poisons and bladder cancer came in 1895 when a German physician tied the high incidence of bladder cancer among workers in the dye industry to the chemicals they were working with. His discovery resulted in laws to protect workers against such exposure. Since then many chemicals have been incriminated as causes of bladder cancer and a number of others are suspected agents.

Here is a list of industrial chemicals which are known to produce bladder cancer in human beings: 2-naphthylamine, benzidine, 4-aminodiphenyl, Chlornaphazine, 2-bis-(2-chloroethyl)-aminonaphthylamine, 1-naphthylamine, Diphenylamine, Auramine, Rosanaline (fuchsin), Dianaisidine, N-1-naphthylthiourea. We are told that there are at present some 1.8 million manmade chemicals at large in the environment and 400 new ones are introduced every year. How many more of these may turn out to be cancer-causing to human beings is anybody's guess at the moment.

Here are other substances now being evaluated for their possible cancer-causing qualities: Pain killers that contain phenacetin, artificial sweeteners, cyclophosphamide and chemicals which interfere with tryptophan metabolism. This is an amino acid or form of protein. Also suspected of being cancer-causing are these: bracken fern, tobacco, viruses and coffee.

Dr. Mount tells us that the incidence of bladder cancer in smokers is approximately twice that of non-smokers. The prospects for recovery are much worse in those who continue smoking than it is in non-smokers or those who have stopped smoking. There seems to be no relationship to cigar or pipe smoking, probably because these smokers do not usually inhale the smoke.

No one knows exactly how tobacco brings about bladder cancer. There may be carcinogenic (cancer-causing) substances in the tobacco smoke itself. This seems to be very likely since arsenic is used to spray the tobacco leaves along with many other pesticides which also may be cancer-causing. Undoubtedly some residue of these poisons remains in the tobacco.

There is also the possibility that the way in which smoking causes bladder cancer is the ability of even one cigarette to lower vitamin C levels in the blood and urine.

"Patients in the bladder tumor population should be advised to stop smoking cigarettes," says Dr. Mount. This is, of course, easier said than done. Surely everyone knows by now that smoking is harmful in many ways, but an increasing number of people are addicted to smoking to such a degree that they find it impossible to stop and maintain any equilibrium in their personal lives.

Dr. Mount says that sufficiently high levels of vitamin C can be obtained in the urine by taking 500 milligrams of vitamin C three times a day at intervals during the day. He quotes Dr. Schlegel of the Tulane University Department of Urology who has been making this recommendation to his bladder patients for many years. Dr. Schlegel practically guarantees that there will be no recurrence of bladder cancer if this prescription is faithfully followed for life.

It is most interesting that cancer patients in general, as well as people "at risk" from bladder cancer and the elderly, as well as smokers, all have low blood levels of vitamin C, says Dr. Mount. Does that not suggest to you an excellent way that all of these groups might fortify themselves against many disorders and possibly prevent cancer—simply by taking enough vitamin C to flood all their tissues with the vitamin?

One and a half grams, which is 1,500 milligrams, taken in three doses throughout the day is completely harmless, says Dr. Mount, and free from the complications which he feels may result from larger doses than that—complications involving oxalic acid in the urine. We would point out that physicians who regularly prescribe much larger doses of vitamin C daily and use these large doses for themselves and their families do not find that the oxalic acid in their urine presents any health problem.

Of course, since Dr. Mount wrote about vitamin C and bladder cancer, we have followed the work of many many practitioners who are regularly prescribing large doses of vitamin C for many conditions, mostly of viral origin. And we have had reports from very reliable sources of terminal cancer patients who were told that no drug therapy could help them. They were sent home to die. Given large amounts of vitamin C by a Scots physician, Dr. Ewan Cameron, many of these patients are still alive and well, with their disease apparently in remission.

Another vitamin mentioned by Dr. Mount as possibly preventive of bladder cancer is vitamin B_6. The vitamin tends to restore the cancer victim's tryptophan metabolism to normal, says Dr. Mount. About half of all patients with bladder cancer excrete elevated amounts of the breakdown products of this amino acid which are believed to be cancer-causing.

Is it possible that some abnormality in the body's use of the amino acid tryptophan may be one cause of bladder cancer? We do not know. But Dr. Mount quotes a famous cancer researcher, Dr. W. C. Hueper, as saying that it is an "unproved but interesting speculation."

Another researcher believes that it is a good case of circumstantial evidence. Dr. Mount says, "It seems reasonable to proceed with a prophylactic (preventive) regimen of 200 milligrams of pyridoxine daily which is non-toxic and may rectify the whole metabolic picture where some cancer-causing chemicals are concerned.

We would point out that the officially recommended daily level of pyridoxine intake is only two milligrams daily, so Dr. Mount is recommending one hundred times this amount. However, it seems reasonable to take extraordinary measures in situations which are extraordinary.

Dr. Mount thinks it may take a long time to arrive at any satisfactory answer to the question of artificial sweeteners and cancer. It would be difficult, he says, to set up an experiment in which one group of human beings taking saccharin is studied in contrast with a control group not taking it, since, he says, at least 75 percent of all Americans have at one time or another taken saccharin.

However, the Ninth National Cancer Conference recommended "in the interim and on the basis of the correlative data presented here, it would appear most prudent at this time to limit utilization of saccharin to diabetics, the severely obese and others with specific medical problems."

Pain killers which contain phenacetin are everywhere. It is an ingredient of most advertised pain remedies and cold remedies. It is advertised for all kinds of not very serious aches and pains like headaches, neuralgias and pain associated with the menstrual cycle. Evidence from Sweden and Australia indicates that there is an increased incidence of bladder cancer among people who use these pain killers to excess.

No one knows for certain that the villain is actually the phenacetin, but its formula is close to that of another chemical known to be cancer-causing. There is also a risk of kidney damage when this drug is used. Dr. Mount says patients "at risk" from bladder cancer should avoid these and all other pain killers.

And now about coffee. A Harvard University researcher was trying to find out more about the relationship of smoking and occupational exposure to chemicals which cause bladder cancer. He found, to his surprise, that there is a greater incidence of bladder cancer among those men and women who drink coffee.

The association of coffee with this kind of cancer was especially strong in the group he studied who did not smoke and were not exposed in their work to industrial substances known to cause bladder cancer.

"This report," says Dr. Mount, "should remind us of the

continuing need to be on the alert to the possibility of carcinogens in our environment."

There is not much comfort for those of us who used to smoke and who smoke no longer. It's well known that cancers sometimes take many years to develop after exposure to the cancer-causing agent. There is not much encouragement in telling ourselves that, well, we don't actually drink that much coffee. It seems likely that people who smoke tend to drink more coffee than non-smokers, since both coffee and cigarettes disrupt blood sugar levels in such a devastating way that the poor victim must reinforce his failing sense of well-being by alternating his props—cigarettes and coffee. If indeed the coffee link to bladder cancer is as strong as that of cigarettes, then this kind of person is most likely to succumb to this extremely disabling and serious condition.

The New York Times for March 27, 1980 reports that a study of more than 2,000 people indicates that working in a roomful of smokers is harmful to nonsmokers, since the smoky air damages the tiny air tubes and sacs in their lungs. The report, written by James R. White and Dr. Herman F. Froeb, measured the effects of on-the-job passive smoking, that is, the fumes people breathe from their neighbors' cigarettes, pipes and cigars. The study took place at the University of California at San Diego.

Mr. White was quoted as saying that, "We know that if a person works around another smoker for a period of time, he will experience lung damage. Now whether it will impair him or cause emphysema, we don't know. But who wants it?"

The *Times* noted that the California study follows a study at Beth Israel Hospital and Harvard University in Boston in 1979 which found poorer lung function in children of parents who smoke. Other studies, the newspaper continued, have suggested that passive smoking can injure the health of non-smoking wives and unborn babies, as well as people with heart and lung diseases and allergies to tobacco smoke.

Although these studies do not link bladder cancer with smoking, it seems possible, does it not, that all of the disorders which affect smokers might eventually affect non-smokers who are continuously exposed to tobacco smoke!

What can the health seeker do to protect himself or herself against this threat? First, obviously, stop smoking if you smoke. Stop smoking if you have to shut yourself up in a room and go "cold turkey" as many other drug addicts must.

It will help greatly if you will, at the same time, break those other harmful habits which contribute to your addiction to smoking. Stop eating sugar or anything that contains it. Eat lots and lots of high protein foods. Eat them at frequent intervals during the day so that you never succumb to that "all-gone" feeling which is one symptom of low blood sugar.

Stop drinking coffee. If you must taper off, it's probably wise to switch to decaffeinated coffee or weak tea, although both, of course contain caffeine, strong tea almost as much as strong coffee. Switch to milk, to fruit juices or to herb teas. But stop drinking coffee.

Don't take pain killers. Most especially don't get into the habit of taking them regularly for any slight headache or joint stiffness. Next time you suffer from any such slight indisposition, go outside and take a long vigorous walk in the fresh air and see if you don't feel better.

And finally get yourself some vitamin C in high potencies and take it every day. If you have been a confirmed smoker and coffee drinker for many years, this expedient becomes even more important. You can perhaps prevent any bladder trouble before it gets started. Get yourself some pyridoxine and take it in the dosages suggested by Dr. Mount and along with some good source of all other B vitamins, since they all work well together.

You can perhaps help to prevent any bladder troubles in the future. In any case, both pyridoxine and vitamin C are harmless in these amounts and may, who knows, bring many other health benefits which you aren't even expecting!

CHAPTER 6

Pyridoxine for Liver and Kidney Disorders

KIDNEY AND LIVER DISEASES are complex, baffling and serious. These organs are essential to body health. Injury to them can bring such a wide variety of disorders, that entire departments of medicine are established to deal just with these two organs.

The liver is the body's chemical factory, its largest organ. Some of its functions are to secrete digestive juices, break down proteins into simpler forms, store blood sugar and fat and release them when needed, maintain correct blood levels of all body compounds and clear foreign matter from the blood.

The kidneys (two of them, one at each side of the body) have the jobs of maintaining the normal water balance of the body, as well as the balance of all body compounds; regulating the concentration of various blood constituents by removing water and certain waste products in the form of urine. Kidneys are small organs, infinitely complex, with millions of tiny filtering units called nephrons. Twice the total blood in a human body is filtered through the kidneys every hour.

Disorders of the liver disrupt almost every body process. Disorders of the kidneys so disrupt the normal flow of wastes from the body that they accumulate in the blood and cause what is called uremic poisoning, which, without heroic medical measures taken to relieve it, can be fatal.

Five scientists working at a veterans hospital in Nashville, Tennessee have been testing the effects of pyridoxine on various diseases. They describe their work on the possible relation of pyridoxine deficiency to uremia and liver disease in the National Academy of Sciences publication, *Human Vitamin B_6 Requirements*.

They first became concerned when they observed that patients with uremia, as well as those with hepatitis (liver inflammation) and heart attacks have abnormal levels of certain compounds in their blood. They had observed, too, that uremic patients suffer from a number of conditions which are similar to those of patients who are deficient in pyridoxine.

These conditions are: depression of the central nervous system, convulsions, changes in skin and mucous membranes, anemia, disorders of the nerves, inability to handle normally the protein in food, increased production of oxalate which may form kidney stones, changes in blood amino acids, depression of the body's ability to resist infections, and low levels of a blood enzyme abbreviated as GOT.

"It seemed possible," say these five scientists, "that some of the problems experienced by the uremic patient might be secondary to a deficiency in vitamin B_6 which accompanies the uremia."

They proceeded to do a number of very complex experiments, testing the amount of pyridoxine in the blood as well as the amounts of the breakdown products of this B vitamin (called PLP) in the blood and in the tissues—products which are intimately involved with how amino acids or proteins are handled by the body.

In every case, the patient with uremia showed abnormal levels of these substances which indicates that these activities are not being carried out normally. One reason why uremia patients are put on low protein diets is that their bodies are not using protein normally, so protein waste products show up in the urine. When the Nashville scientists gave pyridoxine to their uremic patients and to a similar group of healthy people, the uremics were found to have produced only one half as much of the necessary blood compound as the healthy people had produced.

Injecting the essential blood compound into uremic subjects showed that this enzyme was cleared from the blood of these sick people twice as rapidly as it was cleared from the blood of healthy people. Obviously, something was going very wrong in the bodies of the victims of uremia where pyridoxine and its use by the body is concerned.

The authors say, "Such an interference in the activity of a variety of PLP dependent enzymes may occur in other tissues of the body and contribute to the symptoms of the uremic conditions described above."

In the case of liver diseases, PLP (the breakdown product of pyridoxine) is also important. The liver is the primary source of PLP which afterwards appears in the blood. Researchers have shown that chronic alcoholism results in lower levels of PLP in the blood. The Nashville scientists tested patients suffering from three liver disorders—cirrhosis, acute viral hepatitis and extrahepatic obstruction. This is a kind of obstruction related to liver function, but occurring outside the liver itself.

They found that levels of PLP were lower in these sick people. Then they decided to test the effects of injected doses of pyridoxine. They injected 50 milligrams of pyridoxine intravenously in the patients with liver diseases and also in another similar group of healthy men. They found that the pyridoxine in the blood of the patients with liver disease disappeared much more rapidly from the blood than was the case with the healthy people. Apparently the vitamin just wasn't being used normally, so its beneficial effects were rapidly diluted.

The conclusions of the scientists were that there is a vitamin B_6 deficiency state in both uremic patients and in patients with various forms of liver disease. The deficiency

---

Pyridoxine Content of Some Common Foods

(We list milligrams per serving of 100 grams, which is bit more than 3 ounces. Remember that foods like blackstrap molasses and brewers yeast are used in much smaller amounts than this. Even so, their pyridoxine content is remarkable.)

Food	Milligrams of Pyridoxine
Bananas	0.510
Barley	0.220
Beans	0.441
Beef	0.230
Cabbage, raw	0.160
Corn, cooked	0.200
Eggs	0.110
Fish	0.170
Heart, beef	0.250
Kidney, beef	0.430
Lamb	0.275
Liver, beef	0.840
Milk, whole	0.040
Molasses, blackstrap	2.490
Peanuts	0.400
Peas, fresh	0.160
Rice, brown	0.550
Rice, white	0.170
Soybeans	0.810
Wheat bran	0.820
Wheat germ	1.150
Yeast, brewers	2.500

Source: "Home Economics Research Report No. 36, Agricultural Research Service, U.S. Department of Agriculture, Washington, D.C.

seems to be the result of the disease and is a secondary complication of the disease. The patients were on "an adequate diet", say the doctors, so there was no doubt that they were getting what has been assumed to be the required amount of this B vitamin, and there was no evidence that they were not absorbing it. So apparently the deficiency is caused by the rapid disappearance of the breakdown product PLP from the blood, so it cannot be used for all those functions which vitamin B_6 normally fulfills.

The lesson appears to be clear. Give these suffering people more pyridoxine! There is no indication that the doctors proposed doing this, or even suggested that other physicians might try giving pyridoxine to their kidney and liver patients to see if the increased amounts might allow the body to have some spare pyridoxine left so that at least those symptoms which were apparently caused by lack of pyridoxine could be alleviated.

The other aspect of this series of experiments that is disturbing is that the physicians took for granted that the hospital diet contained plenty of pyridoxine for all the patients. They overlooked entirely the fact that individuals have widely varying needs for this vitamin. Doesn't it seem possible that the reason these sick people succumbed to liver and kidney ailments was a simple deficiency in pyridoxine brought about by inherited needs for far larger amounts of the vitamin than any "average" diet could supply?

The total harmlessness of pyridoxine is shown by the fact that it can be injected in 50 milligram doses with no problem of side effects. Why, then, not continue to give it orally or intravenously to everyone suffering from uremia or liver disorders just to see whether lack of this vitamin may be one reason why the patient got the disease? Even if such treatment shows that the disease had other causes (alcoholism, for example) at least some of the most distressing nerve symptoms, perhaps also the anemia and other symptoms which are like those of pyridoxine deficiency might be relieved, giving the patient a more comfortable life.

It seems to us that anyone having early symptoms of any disease condition of the liver or kidneys would do well to make certain he or she is getting plenty of this wholly beneficial vitamin in food and in supplements.

CHAPTER 7

Possible Causes of Multiple Sclerosis

MULTIPLE SCLEROSIS or MS is one of the most common chronic diseases affecting the human brain and spinal cord, reports the National Institutes of Health in 1974. It is characterized by a loss of the fatty sheaths (myelin) that surround the nerve fiber and derives its name from the plaques or patches of scarred (sclerosed) nervous fibers that dot the central nervous system. The government agency estimates that from 100,000 to 250,000 Americans suffer from the disease.

MS advances in a series of unpredictable attacks in most patients, the NIH says. In early stages, attacks are more often followed by periods of remission. With successive episodes, resulting scars in the central nervous system become more numerous, more dense and more destructive, causing progressively severe disability. MS symptoms are not always progressive; some patients experience one or two episodes and are never bothered again.

The cause of multiple sclerosis is unknown. It is, according to an article in *The American Journal of Clinical Nutrition* for August, 1973, probably the most common disease of the central nervous system affecting people between the ages of 20 and 50.

Symptoms of this extremely serious, debilitating disorder include: double vision, nystagmus (uncontrolled rolling of eyeballs), stiffness and weakness of one or more arms or legs, incoordination of muscles, tremor, difficulty in speaking, mental symptoms, emotional instability, convulsive seizures, paralysis of one side of the body, "pins and needles" feelings and difficulties with urination.

Beset by one or more physical and mental problems of this nature at a time when life should be at its fullest, an MS victim is understandably in desperate straits and almost completely at the mercy of the latest medical treatment which never seems to achieve much except to alleviate some symptoms for a while.

Donald A. Mitchell and Emil K. Schandl of Nova University in Florida believe they have found a possible clue to the disease which may prove to be just as helpful to the rest of us as it is to the MS patient. Their theory involves vitamin B_6 and carbon monoxide.

They base their theory on geographical facts and laboratory experiments. They tell us that multiple sclerosis is common only in Western industrialized nations and North America. It is almost unknown in South America, Eastern Europe, North Korea, China, Alaska and the Islands of the Pacific. It rarely appears among African blacks but in the U.S.A. it is as common among blacks as among their white neighbors.

What one environmental factor is present in all those localities where MS is common and not present in other parts of the world? Carbon monoxide pollution of the air, say these authors. It comes from automobile exhausts and from coal-burning chimneys. Carbon monoxide does its damage by attaching itself to hemoglobin, the red coloring matter of blood cells. This results in asphyxiation and death when exposure is maintained long enough. Running a car motor with the garage door closed eventually produces death from carbon monoxide poisoning. Of 21,000 cases of this kind of poisoning who were resuscitated in time, Drs. Mitchell and Schandl tell us, a number suffered a demyelinating condition. This is the same process that causes multiple sclerosis.

Animals exposed to varying amounts of carbon monoxide in the air they breathe exhibit various degrees of destruction of the central nervous system. Left in cages at various highway locations with differing degrees of traffic density, mice were found to have degenerative changes in the nervous system in proportion to the amount of their exposure to carbon monoxide.

Cigarette smoking also brings exposure to carbon monoxide which is in the smoke. More than 50 percent of the smoke in a cigarette may be absorbed by the smoker, and, of course, a smaller amount by anyone in the same room, who is not smoking.

Metal working industries release still more carbon monoxide into outside air. So, for some of us who must travel in heavy traffic, who smoke, who live or work close to polluting industries, exposure to carbon monoxide can be potentially very dangerous.

Now, we come to still another condition that can produce nervous symptoms similar to those of MS. This is deficiency in the B vitamin pyridoxine. In animals, such deficiency produces damage to the spinal cord and the sciatic nerves, stiff hind legs and a peculiar unsteady gait.

Some time ago convulsions were produced in infants fed a commercial formula in which there was no pyridoxine. Some of the infants died before the cause was determined. The incident showed that there may be a forty-fold difference in individual requirements for this B vitamin. That is, someone in your own family or circle of friends may need 40 times more of this vitamin than you need just to be healthy.

Antibiotics and oral contraceptives, as well as several other kinds of drugs, deplete the body of pyridoxine. Since this is a water soluble vitamin, the body's store is easily exhausted. Deficiency in pyridoxine also produces lack of immunity to germs and other toxins. As we have noted, antibodies, which the body makes to protect itself, just cannot be manufactured when not enough pyridoxine is available.

Now we get to the crux of the matter. It has been shown that exposure to carbon monoxide in heavily polluted air increases the body's need for pyridoxine. The researchers who performed these animal experiments warned that, "The use of vitamins in preventing pathophysiologic changes in humans suffering chronic exposure to these gases should be investigated."

Say Mitchell and Schandl, "Assume that a potential MS victim, perhaps a person with a genetically determined higher than usual vitamin B_6 requirement, is exposed to carbon monoxide in his environment over a period of time and that his diet remains relatively unchanged. Under these conditions, even though he is able to maintain an apparently stable level of metabolism, there must be, by logic, a point reached at which the daily intake of pyridoxine will be insufficient to sustain this apparent metabolic need and thus a subjective symptom appears."

The symptom may be determined by what this individual's physical state and need for pyridoxine are.

On the basis of this theory, how can we explain the fact that MS victims sometimes have lengthy remissions when symptoms are less troublesome and nerve tissues seem to be repairing themselves?

Perhaps the exposure to carbon monoxide has lessened, so that requirements for the B vitamin are reduced. Let's say the patient stopped smoking or moved to the country, thus getting away from some of the sources of carbon monoxide which were, theoretically, greatly increasing his need for pyridoxine. Or, let's say his diet was improved to such an extent that he was now getting enough pyridoxine to maintain good nerve function even though he was still exposed to considerable carbon monoxide. In either or both cases, enough pyridoxine might be present to allow the nerve tissues to repair themselves to some extent.

One item of which these scientists seem to be unaware is the fact that pyridoxine is removed from flour and cereals when they are processed and refined into white flour and boxed cereals. Many leading authorities have urged the enrichment of all refined carbohydrates with pyridoxine for this very reason.

It is quite true, also, that in those parts of the world where MS is not prevalent diets are much more likely to be based on *un*refined grains and cereals in which the pyridoxine is intact. So the theory that lack of pyridoxine is part of the cause of MS has still another well-confirmed basis in fact.

Mitchell and Schandl conclude their stimulating article by asking whether it is not possible that those of us who do not succumb to MS may be suffering other nameless, or perhaps well-defined, symptoms relating to our exposure to carbon monoxide and our lack of pyridoxine, even though our symptoms are not so disabling as those of MS victims. We know that cigarette smoking has a deleterious effect on heart health. Is it not possible that the carbon monoxide in the smoke is deleting the body of pyridoxine?

In any case, there is no reason why any of us should sit stupidly, day after day, eating diets deficient in pyridoxine, waiting for nervous symptoms of some kind to strike before we take action. A diet in which there is plenty of pyridoxine is almost certain to be a diet in which other essential nutrients are also plentiful, so it may prevent other nutrition-related disorders as well. A diet in which pyridoxine is lacking is certain to be lacking in many other essential nutrients.

And certainly anyone should be making sure he gets enough pyridoxine by taking some every day in a food supplement—either an all-in-one with high pyridoxine potency or a separate supplement just for pyridoxine. This becomes especially important for anyone exposed to traffic pollution, cigarette pollution, drugs, birth control pills or any of a number of other environmental items which increase our need for pyridoxine.

"From my experience and observation of this 'dread disease,' the tragedy of multiple sclerosis is not that it is an incurable disease but that it is wrongly considered to be one by neurologists, doctors and patients alike. By this I don't mean that it is curable. I know that in the present state of medical knowledge it is not. It is, however, controllable, just as diabetes and celiac disease are. And that is practically as good as a cure."

These are the words of a brilliant and talented Britisher who has won his battle with MS, the crippling disease that strikes mostly young adults, bringing eventual death in many cases. His name is Roger MacDougall. He is a writer, chiefly noted for his screen plays for many movies which have been huge successes in the USA, as well as England. "The Man in the White Suit" is probably his best known movie.

Says MacDougall, "Multiple sclerosis is a name given to an arbitrarily chosen group of symptoms of demyelination. There are many many more symptoms or groups of symptoms of demyelination, or of the condition which causes it, which are given different names. The list is endless," he says. "Paralysis agitans. Transverse myelitis, neuromyelitis, central nervous debility, motor neuron disease, Huntington's Chorea, cerebellar ataxia, scleroderma, dermatomyositis, Friedreich's ataxia, amytrophic lateral sclerosis and many many more.

"It is my deep conviction that these names serve no other purpose than to alarm the unfortunate victim. . . . Multiple sclerosis is a condition which, in my experience,, took a long time to control, though the method of control was comparatively simple. The medical profession, however, is looking for something extremely complicated. The more desperate their fruitless search becomes, the more complexity do they involve in trying to solve the problem."

Doctors cannot solve this disease by looking for one cause, says MacDougall. There is no one cause. Doctors who treat the disease with a low fat diet have discovered only one aspect of the problem. Doctors who prescribe a gluten-free diet are dealing with only one aspect of the problem. MacDougall has found, he says, 17 various pieces of the jig-saw puzzle that is MS. Putting them all together, he has found good health. And so long as he stays on the diet and diet supplements which he developed for himself, he remains well after 17 years of desperate disability. Seventeen years ago he could not see, could not walk, could barely move or talk. Today he is active and touring the country in a crusade to help other MS victims.

Although MacDougall needed many years to arrive at his present controlled condition, he says that much quicker results can be arrived at now, since the full benefits of his diet and diet supplements can be put to work at once. Doctors and researchers who try to test his theories by fragmenting them and testing only this or that part of the therapy will fail, he says. It is the whole therapy which performs the job of enabling the MS victim's body to build new nerve tissue. The therapy does this by first removing from the diet all substances which prevent the building of tissue and by putting into the diet nutrients which encourage cell building.

MacDougall's diet limits or perhaps we should say eliminates as entirely as possible three elements of diet: animal fat, refined white sugar and gluten, a protein in wheat and several other cereals. Cereals which do not contain gluten are permitted. Vegetable fat is permitted. White sugar is forbidden. The diet is difficult to follow unless the patient and his family are willing to go to some lengths to buy and cook special foods.

Bread—regular leavened bread—cannot be made without

gluten. So special gluten-free bread must be bought at the health food store or bread or muffins raised with baking powder must be made at home, *using cereals other than wheat, oats, rye or barley, which are the ones containing gluten.* Rice, corn and millet are permitted, since these cereals contain no gluten. But the restriction of gluten is absolute. No foods may be eaten which contain it. This means checking carefully on every supermarket product to be sure that no trace of any of the four forbidden cereals is present. Any kind of pasta, cakes or other desserts, macaroni, cookies, biscuits, and so on are forbidden. All of them are made commercially from cereals which contain gluten.

Sugar is just as severely restricted. The MS victim may not have any sugar at all, except small amounts of honey or Barbados brown sugar. This means more than just omitting sugar from coffee or tea. All foods containing sugar are forbidden. No desserts but fruit. No sweetened beverages like lemonade or soft drinks. No chewing gum or candy, cakes, doughnuts and so forth.

Animal fat should be cut to a minimum. No butter or cream or fatty cheeses. Use skim milk. Remove all fat from meat. Avoid bacon, sausage, pork and other fatty meats. Use margarine and salad oils for every table and cooking use. These are vegetable fats. Eat the highly nutritious organ meats whenever possible: liver, kidney, heart, tongue, brains. Buy "free-range" animal products whenever you can—eggs from chickens that run free on the farm, meat and poultry from organic farmers who feed their stock in open fields.

Other foods are unrestricted. Vegetables, fruits, nuts, seeds, meat, eggs, yogurt, low fat cheeses like cottage cheese may be eaten in any quantity at any meal. Cereals which do not contain gluten—that is, only millet, rice and corn cereals or breads may be eaten in any quantity. So this is no starvation diet. Only certain foods are limited. Substitutes are available for all these foods.

Instead of animal fat, the MS patient uses mostly vegetable fat in nuts, seeds, margarine and salad oils. Instead of cereals and bread made from the high-gluten cereals (wheat, barley, rye and oats) the MS victim eats bread and cereals made from corn, millet or rice. Instead of sugar, the MS victim eats fruits and vegetables both of which contain lots of natural sugars, plus a bit of honey or brown sugar if he wishes.

Your health food store is the best place to start looking for those cereal foods forbidden on the MacDougall diet. You will find crackers and bread made from millet, rice and corn. Check the label to make certain no wheat, oats, barley or rye is in them. Your health food store has a wide selection of honeys, seeds and nuts, as well as dried fruits and cereals permitted on the MacDougall diet.

Finally, Roger MacDougall takes complete supplements which contain the following nutrients in sizable amounts. His brand is not available in this country, so far as we know, but many brands are available which contain these nutrients, either in separate tablets or in an all-in-one. Or you may prefer a high potency all-in-one, plus some individual capsules or tablets to add to the total.

Here are the recommended vitamins, minerals and other food elements: B_1 (thiamine), B_2 (riboflavin), B_3 (niacin), B_6 (pyridoxine), B_{12}, folic acid, vitamin C, vitamin E, calcium pantothenate, lecithin, magnesium and calcium. Look for these nutrients in tablet form at your health food store. All are beneficial and harmless in reasonable amounts. There is no need to fear overdosage.

For those who are not MS patients, or victims of a related disorder called celiac disease, there is no reason to delete cereals and breads made with the four grains which are rich in gluten: wheat, barley, rye and oats. These are wholesome, nourishing foods for the rest of us who have no problems with gluten. So far as animal fat is concerned, we do not believe that animal fat in reasonable amounts is harmful to the healthy individual. We do recommend cutting fat from meat and choosing lean cuts of meat.

So far as white sugar is concerned, readers of this book should know we believe this to be probably the most pernicious enemy to good health that is available in supermarkets. It seems to us that eliminating white sugar is probably the most important reason for the success of MacDougall's diet. We recommend that all readers delete sugar from their shopping lists as well as all foods that contain it, and see how much better they feel almost at once.

For those who suffer from MS or have an MS victim in their families, you may wish to write to Roger MacDougall for further information about some aspect of his remarkable diet which by now is being used by thousands of people in many parts of the world and, we are told, is bringing relief from this disabling disease. You can reach Roger MacDougall at this address: Regenics, Ltd. 25/27 Oxford St. London W1R 1 RF, England. An airmail stamp for a half-ounce letter costs 31 cents.

There is no need to buy vitamin supplements from England. Exactly the same vitamins and minerals are available in this country. The cost of mailing these products across the Atlantic is very high, chances of their being lost on the way are worrisome. If you wish to follow the MacDougall program in regard to vitamins and minerals, buy them in this country.

CHAPTER 8

Elderly Folks
Don't Get
Enough Pyridoxine

VITAMIN DEFICIENCY is most apt to occur in young children and in old folks. These two groups of our population are also the most vulnerable to diseases of all kinds. So frequent studies are made of the everyday diets of young children and old folks to uncover just what deficiencies they may have and why.

In the case of children, of course, it's the parent's job to provide nourishing diets. But most older folks are on their own when it comes to buying and preparing food. And, unfortunately, it's also their daily job to figure out how to pay for it out of the fixed incomes on which so many older folks are living. As prices rise out of sight, just being able to afford enough food to fill the stomach is a problem, let alone making certain that this food is as nourishing as possible.

Judy Driskell of the Department of Human Nutrition and Foods of Virginia Polytechnic and State University in Blacksburg, Virginia recently conducted a survey of what was actually eaten day after day by 17 elderly men and 20 elderly women living in the vicinity of the University. An interviewer trained to ask questions about diet, food, food buying and preparation, interviewed these 37 people asking for a complete listing of everything they ate in a two-day period.

The object was to discover how much pyridoxine (vitamin B_6) these folks got in their daily meals. And, because pyridoxine is important for guiding the body's use of protein, the amount of protein in the diets was also studied.

The interviewer found that all of the people interviewed got not quite as many calories as the official Recommended Dietary Allowances. They got much more protein and *much less vitamin B_6* than the recommended amount. The actual figures are alarming. Almost half the women and one-fifth of the men reported eating less than 50 percent of the RDA for vitamin B_6. Ninety percent of the women and almost half of the men reported eating less than 70 percent of the RDA for pyridoxine.

These figures are especially significant since they were all eating more protein than the recommended amount, so that their requirement for pyridoxine would be even higher than the recommended amount. Pyridoxine is very much involved with the way our bodies use protein. Every gram of protein food we eat must have its quota of pyridoxine or chances are that things will go wrong somewhere.

Dr. Driskell sought further information on the age of the people interviewed, their incomes, educational levels, food budgets, the preparation of the food, the frequency of "eating out", whether they grew their own vegetables, whether they took vitamin supplements. All these things might influence the findings.

If, for example, they just didn't have enough money to buy nourishing food, that might be the reason for the lack of B_6 in their meals. If they had no knowledge at all about the importance of good nutrition, that might influence their eating habits. And so on. But not one of these things was responsible, apparently, for their lack of pyridoxine.

They were not skimping on food buying. Yes, they knew how to prepare their own food and they did this successfully. Probably those who grew their own vegetables and ate a goodly quantity of them raw had better levels of pyridoxine in their meals than those who ate mostly cooked food, since much pyridoxine is destroyed by cooking.

Testing the blood of these older folks for its pyridoxine content, the scientist found that one third of them had inadequate levels of pyridoxine in their bodies. Those who showed no evidence of any pyridoxine at all in their bodies were found to have diets that varied widely in pyridoxine content. So, says Dr. Driskell, they apparently all have widely varying needs for this vitamin. Perhaps some of those eating the most pyridoxine had none in their bodies, while others eating less pyridoxine did not appear to be deficient in the vitamin.

Only two of the 17 men studied were getting in their meals the full amount—two milligrams of pyridoxine, which is the recommended dietary allowance for this vitamin. Most of the men and women were found to be eating much lower amounts of pyridoxine than that.

The Virginia researcher concludes her study by saying, "Vitamin B$_6$ inadequacy appears to be a nutritional problem in the elderly." We would add that every study we have ever seen of the diets of elderly people shows that they are deficient in most nutrients, not just pyridoxine. And if, as the Virginia study shows, well educated people (who presumably read articles on nutrition and consult their doctors on it, with plenty of money to spend on food and no problems with shopping or cooking their meals or eating out) have this dismal record in regard to such an important item as pyridoxine, what must be the nutritional state of elderly people with much less money who have to scrimp on food buying, who have no facilities for preparing their food or storing their food, who live in apartments, so cannot grow any of their own food?

What was the high protein diet most of these elderly people ate? We have no account of the actual food, but it probably consisted of some eggs and meat, probably also milk and cheese, since these are the foods which contain the most protein. They are also not noted for their pyridoxine content. And if the cereals and breads eaten by the Virginia people were the highly processed kind they contained almost no pyridoxine at all. If nuts and seeds were avoided, with no wheat germ, no bran, no wholegrains, no brown rice, the pyridoxine content of the diet would be very low. Some vegetables are good sources of pyridoxine, but they lose much of it when they are cooked. Raw carrots, cole slaw, tomatoes are fairly good sources of this vitamin, but they should be eaten just about every day. Fruits and berries are poor sources of pyridoxine.

We rather suspect, though we cannot prove it, that the main difficulty with the diets of these elderly people was their reliance on processed cereals and breads, rather than wholegrain ones. We are told that such depleted foods, along with sugar, make up half the diets eaten by most Americans, which means we must have an almost universal deficiency in pyridoxine. And, we suspect, this deficiency is probably much more prevalent and much more serious in elderly folks.

CHAPTER 9

Dealing with Nausea and a Hangover

LAWRENCE GALTON describes nausea as something that verges on being indescribable. It is a sick feeling, a tightness in the throat, he says, a sinking sensation and a feeling that one is soon going to vomit. Often vomiting does follow, along with paleness, faintness, weakness and a racing pulse.

"Morning sickness" of pregnancy involves nausea. So does motion sickness. Emotional disturbances often trigger it, or intense pain. And food poisoning of several kinds causes nausea and vomiting. Both are supposed to occur because the stomach does not want any more food. And surely, the last thing the nauseated person wants to do is eat. It is believed that the nausea is brought about to prevent eating so that the digestive tract can get into good shape again before being forced to deal with more food. And vomiting to get rid of whatever food is there in the stomach means that some of it is possibly poisonous.

For many years doctors have been treating morning sickness with pyridoxine. As doctor after doctor discovers this treatment, he generally rushes into print to describe this easy, inexpensive and harmless way of relieving one of life's greatest miseries, nausea.

Most recently an Austrian physician tested a number of

pregnant women suffering from the nausea of morning sickness and found they were deficient in vitamin B_6. He gave them 200 milligrams of the vitamin daily for a week, then five milligrams daily thereafter and cured nausea.

William H. Sebrell, Jr., M.D., in the massive work *Vitamins and Hormones*, volume 22, 1964, reported that "Vitamin B_6 has been used clinically on an empirical basis in the treatment of nausea and vomiting during the first trimester (three months) of pregnancy. . . . it would appear that pregnancy either alters vitamin B_6 metabolism or increases the demand so that the requirement during pregnancy is higher than usual creating a need that is not being met by dietary intake of some pregnant women."

Dr. John M. Ellis in his fine book, *Vitamin B_6, the Doctor's Report*, states that "radiologists used B_6 to some extent in an effort to relieve nausea associated with deep X-ray therapy in the treatment of cancer. Meanwhile obstetricians claimed some success in treating nausea of pregnancy with B_6. . . ."

Carlton Fredericks, in his book *The Nutrition Handbook, Your Key to Good Health* says, "This is one of the most promising of all the vitamins and it is almost certain that continuing research will discover more marvels than are now known. It has already been seen to accomplish near-miracles—restoring function to paralyzed legs (where nerves were involved in the pathology); shrinking enlarged hearts, and relieving distressed intestinal tracts after a lifetime of misery for dyspepsia sufferers. Doctors have reported that pellagra patients do not recover their full strength until given vitamin B_6. Surgeons administer the vitamin before operating to avoid post-operative nausea from ether and many obstetricians find that the nausea of pregnancy can sometimes be interrupted with vitamin B_6."

Adelle Davis in *Let's Get Well*, says, "Burning sensations in the mouth may be the first symptoms of a vitamin B_6

deficiency. . . . Both nausea and vomiting have been produced in persons deficient in magnesium or vitamin B_6; and the latter deficiency is accompanied by butterflies and burning pain in the stomach, bloating, abdominal soreness and cramps, and the passing of excessive amounts of gas both orally and rectally. Conversely, vitamin B_6 has been used successfully to stop the vomiting of pregnancy and of car, sea, air and radiation sickness."

Merck Manual, the doctors' bible where treatment is concerned, has this to say about morning sickness.

"Most patients with morning sickness respond to reassurance and small dry meals, fluids being taken between meals. Eating a cracker before getting out of bed and avoiding excess fluid intake may prevent nausea. If possible, drugs should be avoided because of possible teratogenic effects. . . . Pyridoxine 50 to 100 milligrams intramuscularly or orally has been valuable in some cases."

Nausea which appears out of nowhere for no apparent reason and persists should, of course, be diagnosed by a physician or possibly an ophthalmologist. Many eye conditions or incorrect eyeglass prescriptions can produce devastating nausea. If this does not disappear as one grows accustomed to the glasses, it's time to see if changes can't be made.

Meanwhile there is nothing to prevent you from making certain you are getting enough pyridoxine, no matter what the cause for nausea may be. There is general agreement among many top nutrition experts that we are not getting enough in our meals, especially since many of us may have greatly increased needs for this vitamin. Refined carbohydrates, (white flour, white sugar and processed cereals) which make up so large a part of most modern diets, are all devoid of this essential nutrient which must be present in ample quantities for normal digestion of all proteins, fats and carbohydrates.

Recently chemists at a West German drug company made some changes in the chemical formula of vitamin B_6 and found that it seemed to prevent symptoms of intoxication in their laboratory animals. They did further studies and reported on them in scientific journals.

Several physicians in Denmark decided they would try the pyridoxine compound on some human volunteers to see if it worked with them. It appeared to be harmless, so there was no reason not to make the experiment.

They enlisted the aid of 11 men and six women, all healthy, who volunteered to come to planned parties and drink all they wanted to drink of any kind of booze that appealed to them. For five hours they socialized getting a little "higher" all the time. Pills had been distributed to each of them at the beginning of the parties. Some of the pills contained the new derivative of pyridoxine. Others contained nothing but filler.

After the parties were over, the volunteers were checked for hangover symptoms. These might include vomiting, heartburn, lassitude, overwhelming thirst, palpitations of the heart, weakness of joints, giddiness and dizziness, headache, sweating, pallor, depression, inability to walk a straight line, and a general feeling of discomfort.

Checking with the carefully kept secret records as to who had the pyridoxine and who had the "nothing" pill, the Danish doctors found that symptoms like those listed above were minimized in the volunteers who got the pill containing the pyridoxine compound. Not completely eliminated, but made much less agonizing.

For example, some of the volunteers had complete amnesia for everything that happened at the parties. Alcoholics know this feeling well. It's as if they had blacked out when the party started. When they are told the next day what they did and said at the party, they refuse to believe it.

Those volunteers who got the B vitamin pill had no amnesia the next day. They remembered everything that happened. Furthermore their speech was not slurred as was the speech of some of those who got the "nothing" pill rather than the B vitamin.

The work of the Danish doctors was published in the *Quarterly Journal of Studies of Alcoholism*, volume 34, page 1195, 1973. We don't know of any source of the particular pyridoxine compound which was used, but there seems to be no reason not to use the regular B_6 tablet which is inexpensively available at any health food store. It's safe to take B_6 in even very large amounts unless you happen to have a worrisome stomach ulcer, in which case you might have to be a little more careful, for the vitamin seems to increase the amount of stomach acid, or digestive juice.

The best thing to do about drinking, of course, is to stop, gradually, if that's the easiest way for you to do it. It has been known for many years that alcohol depletes the body of B vitamins, as sugar does, since both are substances containing no B vitamins whatsoever, but needing large amounts of them in order for the body to process the sugar or the alcohol.

As all drinkers know, it's always best to eat at the same time you are drinking, so that you never drink on an empty stomach. It's best never to drink alone. It's best never to "need" a drink at any special time of day. And it's best to stop drinking entirely if you would be healthy.

Meanwhile, and for those occasions when you may have to drink or be impolite, (the toasts at a friend's wedding, for instance) remember to load up on pyridoxine beforehand, so that there will be no chance of a serious and painful hangover if you get carried away and drink a bit more than you intended to.

CHAPTER 10

Early Arthritis Symptoms and a B Vitamin

HERE ARE SOME of the conditions that are commonly found in living creatures that are deficient in vitamin B_6: in the monkey, lack of pyridoxine brings on hardening of the arteries. In rats a condition called acrodynia results. The medical dictionary defines this as a condition usually of infants marked by extreme irritability, alternating with periods of apathy, lack of appetite, pink itching hands and feet, fear of light, profuse sweating, rapid heart beat, high blood pressure, and several other symptoms. It is associated, says the dictionary, usually with mercury poisoning, but it may also be present "with inflammatory changes of obscure origin in the central nervous system." The dictionary does not mention lack of vitamin B_6

In human beings lack of vitamin B_6 may bring on a reduction in the amount of lymph in the body, convulsions, dermatitis, irritability and nervous disorders.

That's quite a catalog of misery. But strangely enough, perceptive, innovative physicians keep turning up still more disorders which are apparently related to lack of this important B vitamin, or at any rate, disorders which respond to the administration of quite large doses of the B vitamins.

Early symptoms of arthritis appear to be conditions of this kind, according to Dr. John Ellis, a Texas physician who has specialized in the use of pyridoxine for many mysterious conditions that would yield to no other therapy.

Dr. Ellis began his use of vitamin B6 when he noticed that patients complained of trouble with their hands. There is a numbness or tingling of hands and fingers. The little finger may be the first to become involved, he says. The patient may complain that his hands "go to sleep" when he is in bed at night. Fingers may become stiff so that it is almost impossible to "make a fist." There is pain in the joints and the grip becomes so weak that things are easily dropped.

The hands may swell, then, so that rings become too tight. At night an entire arm may appear to be paralyzed, so that the other arm must be used to shake it "awake." The sense of touch may be affected so that, with eyes closed, the patient cannot tell the difference in texture between glass and rough wood. "Charley horse" or leg cramps may be very troublesome at night, while the patient vainly tries to massage the cramping leg back to some degree of comfort.

Little knots or bumps may appear at the side of fingers. Doctors call these "Heberden's Nodes", named after the English physician who first described this condition. Then arms and shoulders may be affected. Pain may be located in the shoulder, below it or in the arm between the shoulder and elbow. Questioned about his condition, the patient will probably say, "I have rheumatism."

Dr. Ellis, in a chapter in the massive book *A Physician's Handbook on Orthomolecular Medicine*, says, about this condition, "The people studied in Northeast Texas, and there were hundreds, perhaps thousands that I saw, did have rheumatism and they exhibited spectacular response to vitamin B6 given 50 milligrams daily by mouth. . . . There are dozens of patients in Northeast Texas who have taken pyridoxine 50 milligrams daily for eight years, and there are thousands who have taken pyridoxine 50 milligrams daily for the last four years."

He goes on to say, "Motion pictures, taken before and after treatment with pyridoxine have objective proof that vitamin B_6 reduced swelling in hands and fingers, improved range of finger flexion, improved speed of finger flexion, improved coordination of finger movement, prevented transitory nocturnal arm paralysis, and halted night time leg cramps and muscle spasms.

"Subjectively, after six weeks of therapy, there was improvement of sensation and perception in finger tips, and there was elimination of numbness and tingling in hands and fingers. Shoulder pain was reduced or eliminated and shoulder and arm function was improved. Finger joints that had been tender and painful before treatment were substantially improved after six weeks of therapy with pyridoxine."

Dr. Ellis relates his experiences in giving pyridoxine in doses up to 300 milligrams daily to pregnant women and reducing dramatically the painful swelling in their hands and feet—and all this without any reduction of salt in their diets and without diuretics or "water pills."

It is well known that The Pill, the oral contraceptive, destroys pyridoxine in the body of many women who take The Pill. Such serious deficiencies have been found in many women on The Pill that some physicians have asked that all oral contraceptives carry a dose of pyridoxine in the same pill. This suggestion has been ignored by both the Food and Drug Administration and the makers of The Pill.

Doesn't it seem possible that many of the troubles with edema or swelling of hands and feet in pregnant women who have been on The Pill may be caused by lack of this vitamin?

"Onset of the disease syndrome known as rheumatism was gradual (among his patients)," says Dr. Ellis. "There was edema of hands and fingers long before there was experience of pain and stiffness in shoulders. Occasionally, there was a rather sudden onset of signs and symptoms that has been alluded to as the 'shoulder-hand-syndrome'. The long standing cases were more difficult to relieve, and ordinarily the older-aged people had less response to pyridoxine. There was no doubt, however, that patients with the 'shoulder-hand-syndrome' exhibited improvement of hand function, reduction of edema (swelling) and moderate relief of pain in shoulders when pyridoxine was given 50-100 milligrams daily for six weeks. Reduction of edema and improvement in hand function could be observed within one week of initiation of treatment."

Dr. Ellis is quick to point out that other nutrients are important, too. Pyridoxine is not a "miracle drug" that can guarantee instant relief of pain and swelling if an atrocious diet is eaten and all other vitamins (especially B complex vitamins) are ignored.

Dr. Ellis suggests wheat germ as an excellent source of pyridoxine. Brewers yeast, too, is a good source, though not so tasty, so a bit more difficult to work into one's diet. Leafy vegetables—the dark green ones like spinach and watercress, turnip greens and broccoli—are also good sources of pyridoxine, as well as other B vitamins and many minerals and trace minerals.

Most important of all, one should avoid those foods from which the pyridoxine and most other nutrients have been removed, for these foods present your body with a dilemma that it cannot solve and remain healthy. The foods we mean are white sugar and white flour and every food made from them. They contain relatively huge amounts of carbohydrates from which practically all the B vitamins, the minerals and trace minerals have been removed in the refining process. These B vitamins, and the minerals and trace minerals as well, (chromium, for example) are absolutely essential for your body to use the carbohydrates healthfully. So by avoiding these foods, you are, in a manner of speaking, saving pyridoxine and other B vitamins.

When all these essential nutrients are lacking—and they are lacking in the average American diet loaded with sugar and white bread—things are bound to go wrong, healthwise. Widespread incidence of arthritis and rheumatism is apparently one of the penalties we pay for not recognizing this fact and for continuing to buy and eat these staple, popular foods.

You can feel perfectly safe in taking large amounts of pyridoxine—even larger amounts than Dr. Ellis gave his patients. Like all other B vitamins, it is water soluble, so whatever is not used is rather quickly excreted. It is not stored in the body to any great extent. By the same token, you should take all the B vitamins, including pyridoxine, rather frequently during the day to get the best effect.

Don't decide that a few hundred milligrams once a week or once a month will accomplish anything much. And don't take all your B vitamins at breakfast and forget them for the rest of the day. It's always a good idea to space the B vitamins and vitamin C so that you take small amounts of them at every meal—three times a day. If you happen to be one of those individuals who needs large amounts of pyridoxine or other B vitamins then you need large amounts every day, not just occasionally when you remember to take them.

Dr. Ellis feels that there is only one precaution about taking large doses of pyridoxine. There is some evidence, he says, that this B vitamin "has something to do with histamine production and very likely it increases production or action of stomach secretions. At any rate, people who have stomach ulcers should be under treatment before beginning use of vitamin B_6." By this we suppose he means large doses of B_6, for everybody who takes even a one-a-day vitamin tablet is getting some pyridoxine in it. Large doses of any vitamin or mineral should probably be taken with or directly after meals, for the same reasons that drugs cause least problems taken this way. You should not pour a powerful substance into an empty stomach. The food helps to dilute the vitamin and the vitamin is metabolized most effectively with the food in which it occurs naturally.

For women on The Pill it is necessary to take pyridoxine every day along with the many other nutrients that this hormone drug destroys in the body. The Pill is creating a condition of pregnancy in the woman's body every month. All the extraordinary measures that the body calls into play to conduct a successful pregnancy are called upon. Then The Pill is stopped for a period of menstruation, and the body's elaborate preparations for pregnancy are stalled. The next month the same cycle takes place. No wonder essential nutrients are wasted and disappear from the body creating deficiencies whose full destructive power may not be demonstrated for many years to come.

Pyridoxine is one of these nutrients. It also seems to be deficient in people who are just beginning to notice the advance of arthritic symptoms. Replacing it by taking a daily supplement is only common sense. Since no one knows how much any individual may need of this B vitamin, it's best to be safe rather than sorry. Taking more of the B vitamins than you may need is insurance, the best kind of health insurance there is.

Dr. Roger J. Williams in his excellent book, *Nutrition Against Disease*, has this to say about the collagen diseases, arthritis and related disorders: "While medical education has put a damper on experiments in which the nutrition of arthritics might have been studied and manipulated in an expert fashion, there is excellent reason for thinking that if this were done, sufferers could get real rather than palliative relief. There is even a good possibility that individual arthritics will be able—if they are lucky and make intelligent trials—to hit upon particular nutrients or nutrient combinations which will bring relief.

". . . On the basis of reports presently available, the items that certainly need to be considered are niacin (niacinamide), pantothenic acid, riboflavin, vitamin A, vitamin B_6, vitamin C, magnesium, calcium, phosphate and other minerals. The objective is to feed *adequately* the cells that are involved in keeping the bones, joints and muscles in healthy condition."

Dr. Williams refers back to one of his favorite themes: biological individuality. Each of us has his own characteristic nutritional needs for various nutrients. They remain with us through life. Those with back and neck pain throughout life may simply be suffering from lack of enough vitamin C since their needs may be higher than the average person's.

"I certainly would not want to give the impression that the management of these diseases is simple," says Dr. Williams. "But I do reaffirm the dictum that nutrition should be tried first. On the basis of reports presently available, the items that certainly need to be considered are niacin (vitamin B_3), pantothenic acid, riboflavin (vitamin B_2), vitamin A, vitamin B_6 (pyridoxine), vitamin C, magnesium, calcium, phosphate (phosphorus) and other minerals. The objective is to feed adequately the cells that are involved in producing synovial fluid and in keeping bones, joints and muscles in healthy condition."

Dr. Williams' wise recommendations on arthritis make up one chapter in his fine book, wherein this distinguished nutrition researcher recommends what he calls "supernutrition"—a condition, he says, which no living being on the earth has yet experienced—including human beings.

In a book published in 1949, *The Common Form of Joint Dysfunction: Its Incidence and Treatment*, the late Dr. William Kaufman describes how he used vitamin B_3 (niacin) and other vitamins in rather large doses to treat arthritis. In most cases he also gave quite large doses of vitamin B_6, vitamin C, vitamin B_1 and vitamin B_2. He tailored the dosage of vitamin B_3 (in this case, niacinamide) according to the individual patient's needs. If there appeared to be little or no improvement, he increased the dosage. If improvement appeared to have stopped at a "plateau," he increased the dosage. He cautioned his patients to continue with the recommended dosage even if they became discouraged with slow progress. Improvement with this completely harmless therapy appears to take quite a long time, although in several cases described in the book almost miraculous improvement occurred in a matter of months in people who had suffered for years from arthritis.

Dr. Kaufman's work with vitamin B_3 is discussed in more detail in *Arthritis*, by Ruth Adams and Frank Murray, published in 1979 by Larchmont Books.

CHAPTER 11

Can Pyridoxine Help Prevent Diabetes?

"Vitamin B_6 therapy may be a link in the prevention of diabetes as well as a number of other diseases," says Dr. John Ellis in his book *Vitamin B_6: the Doctor's Report.*

"In my own practice I have seen a relationship between the two that provides clinical clues in this direction. Many diabetics have turned up with signs and symptoms that, in other patients, were successfully treated with B_6. In turn, the diabetic so suffering also benefited. Many patients with diabetes mellitus had disturbed tactile (touch) sensations in their fingers that responded to pyridoxine. Furthermore, I have noted that most elderly diabetics have edema in their hands and fingers. These conditions responded favorably to 50 milligrams of pyridoxine daily."

Dr. Ellis tells us also of a Japanese laboratory researcher, Yakito Kotake, who worked with animals in establishing a link between pyridoxine and diabetes.

His theory goes like this. A certain amino acid or form of protein called tryptophan is broken down in the body into the B vitamin niacin, if this process is normal. Pyridoxine is necessary for this process "as it is for every other amino acid studied," says Dr. Ellis. If enough pyridoxine is not present, a certain acid will be excreted in the urine, indicating that the processing of the amino acid was not normal due to lack of this B vitamin. Kotake has found that this acid is invariably present in the urine of diabetics, indicating that the entire process is disturbed due to lack of the B vitamin.

Kotake has also found that this acid (xanthurenic acid) is a cause of diabetes. Through a complicated process it results in the exhaustion of cells in the pancreas. And diabetes is a disorder of pancreatic function.

"Of course," says Dr. Ellis, "complete destruction of these particular cells in the pancreas cannot be reversed by pyridoxine but Kotake has demonstrated that pyridoxine will prevent all manifestation of the diabetogenic (diabetes-causing) effect of xanthurenic acid."

He tells the story of his patient with diabetes and advanced hardening of the arteries whose hands were swollen and who had cramps in his legs when he walked. The sensation of touch in his fingertips had also degenerated until he could not feel the weave in a tablecloth.

With nothing more than 50 milligrams of pyridoxine daily, and without changing the patient's diet or giving him any other treatment for diabetes, Dr. Ellis restored his sense of touch and cured the swelling in his hands and fingers. When this patient went to a hospital later on for circulatory complications, he took no pyridoxine for the seven weeks he was there. All the complaints returned. He could not hold the steering wheel of his car without his hands going to sleep. Once home, he began to take 50 to 100 milligrams of pyridoxine daily and, once again, the symptoms disappeared.

Writing in the September, 1974 issue of *National Food and Farming*, Dr. Ellis said that a British scientist has shown that women taking The Pill have abnormal excretion of xanthurenic acid, indicating a tendency toward diabetes. The oral contraceptive depletes the body of pyridoxine in many women who take it.

Dr. David Rose at St. Mary's Hospital in London showed

that The Pill given to 31 women caused abnormal blood sugar levels in 12 of them. Forty milligrams of pyridoxine given to the women daily lowered the high blood sugar levels to normal.

"It must be emphasized," says Dr. Ellis, "that many scientific papers have indicated that it is the estrogen (female hormone) in birth control pills that is causing the different complications of high blood pressure, sugar intolerance and elevated triglyceride (fat) and cholesterol levels. It should also be emphasized that women who are taking estrogen in the postmenopausal state are in the same jeopardy as are the younger women who are taking estrogen in birth control pills."

Dr. Ellis has often been asked, he says, how prevalent is vitamin B$_6$ deficiency. He believes this is best answered by listing those conditions in which large doses of the B vitamin appear to improve the health. He has successfully treated hundreds of people with rheumatism of hands, shoulders and arms with 50 to 100 milligrams of pyridoxine daily.

It is common knowledge, he says, that in the United States and England one-third of all pregnant women suffer from edema of pregnancy in which there are gross collections of fluid with swollen hands and feet. He has found, he says, that 50-400 milligrams of pyridoxine daily will produce marked reduction in this swelling *within 72 hours*.

Arthritis with severe pain, numbness and tingling hands and fingers of women of about 40 years of age can be relieved with 50 to 100 milligrams of pyridoxine. Men complaining of the same middle-age symptoms may also be suffering from effects of the female hormone, since this hormone is also present to some degree in the male. "Many times I have seen swelling in the hands of heart patients relieved by vitamin B$_6$," says Dr. Ellis.

"So if one totals . . . the millions of people with rheumatism, those with menopausal arthritis, one-third of the pregnant population, those with arteriosclerosis (hardening of the arteries) and heart attacks, those with diabetes, and finally adds the eight million women who use birth control pills, it is reasonable to state that either pyridoxine deficiency or greatly increased need for pyridoxine very likely constitute the most serious and most prevalent nutrition derangement in the United States. . . . My documentation is based on case histories of hundreds of patients, many of whom I have observed for 10 years and who have been taking 50-100 milligrams of pyridoxine daily for ten years without any ill effect."

Dr. Ellis lists the following conditions in which pyridoxine will probably be helpful: The shoulder-hand syndrome (numbness, tingling and pain); the carpal tunnel syndrome (swelling, numbness and pain in hands and wrists); premenstrual tension; idiopathic edema (swelling of unknown origin); pregnancy; menopausal arthritis; diabetes mellitus; mental retardation, including convulsion. Lasting mental retardation results from sustained vitamin B_6 deficiency, says Dr. Ellis. He also believes that some sufferers from lupus erythematosus and scleroderma may respond to large doses of pyridoxine.

The American Journal of Obstetrics and Gynecology (March 1, 1977) reported on thirteen women in late pregnancy who developed diabetes. Each of them was given 100 milligrams of vitamin B_6 daily for two weeks. Blood sugar levels tested again showed marked reduction of blood sugar levels. "These results suggest that a relative deficiency in vitamin B_6 is associated with some cases of gestational (pregnancy) diabetes and that the replacement of this vitamin improves the metabolic state," says Dr. W. N. Spellacy of the Florida College of Medicine.

An editorial in the April 10, 1976 issue of the British medical journal *The Lancet*, speculates on just what the mechanism of vitamin B_6 is in lowering blood sugar levels in diabetics. Diabetic women who are pregnant and women taking The Pill are considered at risk of chronic diabetes which may be prevented if enough vitamin B_6 is given. It's possible, says the editorial, that diabetes in pregnant women may be partly brought about by an inherited tendency toward high blood sugar, but there seems to be lots of evidence that lack of pyridoxine is at least partly responsible.

An April 26, 1976 issue of *The Lancet* describes tests with 46 women taking The Pill, all of whom had abnormal processing of the amino acid tryptophan, suggesting that the B vitamin pyridoxine was not functioning normally even though only 18 women seemed to have a deficiency of the vitamin in their blood. In some of the women with vitamin B_6 deficiency there were indications of disorders in sugar metabolism, suggesting a tendency to diabetes.

There are three very important reasons why pyridoxine deficiency may be incapacitating many more Americans than is generally realized.

First, Almost all of the pyridoxine is removed when grains are refined and processed into white flour and supermarket cereals. The vitamin is not restored in the bread "enrichment" program. We get some of only three of the B vitamins restored—but no pyridoxine.

Second, diets high in fat and protein make our needs for pyridoxine higher. American diets are high in protein and fat. Fast food meals are loaded with the fat from fried or grilled fatty meats and french fries as well as the ice cream and milk shakes that generally accompany them. Heaps of whipped cream on desserts which may already be half fat add to the fat content of our meals. With every gram of fat we eat our requirement for pyridoxine increases.

Third, it is true of all vitamins, but of pyridoxine especially, that individual needs may vary enormously. In 1952 many babies getting commercial formulas that were deficient in pyridoxine developed convulsions. Some of these infants died. Others had serious convulsions but survived. Others had no convulsions. This seems to indicate that the individual needs of the babies for this vitamin varied so widely that the variations could mean the difference between life and death.

There appears to be much evidence that an inherited tendency toward blood sugar disorders like diabetes may also indicate a great need for large doses of pyridoxine. There is also much evidence that one individual may need much more pyridoxine than another to overcome this tendency. And there is overwhelming evidence that most of us are just not getting enough pyridoxine in our meals.

CHAPTER 12

Pyridoxine and a Mysterious Disorder of the Wrist

CARPAL TUNNEL SYNDROME is a painful disorder of the wrist. It involves the nerve which passes through the "tunnel" formed by the eight bones of the wrist. The nerve is compressed, resulting in peculiar disturbances of sensation in that area of the skin which this nerve enters. There is pain when the wrist is bent, fingers may be swollen, the skin on the hands is stretched and shiny.

In his book *Vitamin B₆, the Doctor's Report*, Dr. John M. Ellis tells us that diagnosis of this complaint is based on three major things that are wrong. There is impaired feeling in the hand and wrist. There is a tingling sensation in the wrist that radiates out into the hand. A test can be performed which will clinch the diagnosis.

"I have given a prominent position in this chapter to the carpal tunnel syndrome," says Dr. Ellis, "because of the attention the medical literature has been giving it in relatively recent years. For nearly a century now the literature has discussed paresthesia of the hands. (The medical dictionary defines this term as "a perverted sensation of tingling, crawling or burning of the skin.") During more recent times the orthopedic surgeons have shown that much of this paresthesia of the hands was a spontaneous compression of the median nerve (of the wrist)."

Dr. Ellis says that the hands of many people with this condition are swollen, both on the back and palm of the hands. "The carpal tunnel syndrome is inseparably associated with a hormone and (vitamin) B_6 relationship. The carpal tunnel syndrome appears during pregnancy, with the use of the birth control pill and more frequently in persons who have a family history of diabetes."

The symptoms of this condition were described in medical literature as long ago as 1880. Pains in the shoulders and arms often accompany it. So it is apparently associated with arthritis. Since the condition is three times more common in women than in men, it is believed that disorders of sex hormones must play some part in it. It has been treated mostly with surgery.

The doctor who has done the most research on this subject in the past, George S. Phalen, has described chronic inflammation and thickening of fibrous material in the area which would compress the nerve. This doctor also pointed out, in a study of 439 patients, that 27.2 percent either had diabetes or a history of diabetes in the family. Other disorders sometimes found with this one are "trigger finger" (a condition in which a finger cannot be bent or straightened except in a jerky movement), "trigger thumb", rheumatoid arthritis and "tennis elbow."

As he was studying these facts in the pages of medical journals, Dr. Ellis became aware, he tells us, that symptoms of many of his patients were in fact carpal tunnel syndrome.

"During the preceding years," he says, "I had learned that pyridoxine would relieve premenstrual edema, the edema of pregnancy, menopausal arthritis and the edema (swelling) associated with the use of anti-ovulatory hormones (birth control pills)."

During the period from 1962 to 1972, Dr. Ellis treated about 225 pregnant patients with pyridoxine. All suffered from swollen feet and/or hands. They all had symptoms much like those of the carpal tunnel syndrome—numbness and tingling in fingers and hands, especially at night, weakness of hand grip, a tendency to drop objects, swollen hands and fingers.

Dr. Ellis developed a test by which he could measure the improvement which the vitamin B_6 brought. The test is this. Hold the hands out with palms up. Now bend the fingers at the two outer joints only, leaving the knuckle joints in a straight line with the wrists. Bring the tips of the fingers down to the palms of the hands, right to the crease that separates fingers from hands. The knuckle joints must remain straight throughout. Do not make a fist, for that means you are bending the knuckle joints. These must remain straight. The object of the test is to discover whether the fingertips can touch the palm of the hand without bending the knuckles.

If any one of these 16 joints cannot be bent completely and without pain (unless you have had fractures or other injuries or infections) then you probably need additional vitamin B_6. Dr. Ellis gave the test to older patients with arthritis and he was generally successful in relieving the condition if the arthritis had not been present for too many years. "Usually, however," he says, "age did not hamper the beneficial effects of B_6.

Dr. Ellis gives us some case histories. A 33-year-old typist complained that her right hand had suddenly become weak so that she would drop objects, especially heavy objects. Her hand felt "asleep" or numb. Her hand would wake her at night, her fingers swelled, so that rings could not be removed. She had been taking The Pill for ten years, and for six years had taken no vitamin supplements of any kind. She also had cold perspiration on the palm of the right hand.

Dr. Ellis gave her an injection of 50 milligrams of pyridoxine and told her to take 50 milligrams at night and in the morning every day. Within one week most of the symptoms had subsided. Some six weeks later she had no pain, tingling or swelling. She continued to take The Pill.

A 21-year-old woman who was pregnant was relieved of swelling of hands and feet and pain in fingers when she took varying amounts of pyridoxine during her pregnancy. Three years later she developed severe pain in her right hand, arm and shoulder. Fifty milligrams of pyridoxine three times a day eliminated the pain. All pain, swelling and the movement of her hands returned to normal.

Aside from Dr. Ellis a number of researchers have reported the occurrence of carpal tunnel syndrome in pregnancy and while taking The Pill. In some of these latter women, just discontinuing The Pill eliminated the symptoms. When they started to take it once again the pain, weakness and tingling returned.

"Thus," says Dr. Ellis, "we have a manifold increase in estrogen (the female sex hormone) and other hormones during pregnancy, and anti-ovulatory pills (birth control pills) also account for an increase in estrogen. In turn, estrogen causes derangement in excretion of the same metabolites associated with B_6 deficiency. From this it follows that during these two times of life, certainly, the diet should be supplemented with B_6, for the carpal tunnel syndrome as associated with pregnancy and with contraceptive pills does respond to large doses of pyridoxine."

In a recent issue of the *American Journal of Clinical Nutrition*, (October, 1979), Dr. Ellis and a group of researchers from Texas tested the vitamin on a patient who had suffered from carpal tunnel syndrome for many months. Pain pills, tranquilizers and sleeping pills had made no difference. Every night was agony because of the pain as well as the numbness and tingling in his wrists and the palms of his hands.

The Texas researchers remind us of previous experiences of Dr. Ellis in which he gave pyridoxine in massive doses to 21 patients who had been shown to be deficient in pyridoxine. It took up to 11 weeks of treatment with 300 milligrams of this vitamin daily to correct the condition and cure the pain. Dr. Ellis succeeded in doing it. The official recommended daily allowance for vitamin B_6 is 2 milligrams. So it's very obvious that all these folks were dreadfully deficient in the vitamin and had to build up stores of it over a long time before it finally produced the effects they were seeking. It did not accomplish this overnight. It is well to keep this fact in mind when you are using one or more vitamins to treat a disorder.

The Texas doctors tested the patient described above and found that he was indeed deficient in pyridoxine. This should not be unexpected since his diet almost guaranteed such a deficiency. He ate no breakfast, had meat sandwiches, candy and a soft drink for lunch, vegetables and beans along with some small amount of meat for dinner. Not much pyridoxine there.

The patient was given two milligrams of pyridoxine for nine weeks and noticed considerable improvement in the condition of his wrists and fingers. After two more weeks there was a bit more improvement. But the patient's hands were not nearly normal yet. He was then given 100 milligrams of pyridoxine for 11 more weeks with more improvement in some joints.

A "placebo" was then substituted for the pyridoxine. This is a pill which looks just like the one being tested, but contains nothing. The patient did not know that he was no longer getting the pyridoxine which had brought great improvement. Gradually, as he was taking the "nothing" pill, the painful condition returned and measurements showed that his vitamin B_6 deficiency had also returned. Obviously he needed to take a pyridoxine supplement all the time to make up for the pyridoxine he was not getting in meals. Doctors began again to use the real pill, the pyridoxine, and his condition gradually improved until it was once again normal. They tried the placebo again and his condition degenerated gradually while his deficiency in vitamin B₆ returned. The doctors point out that this patient had been in such pain that he could not sleep for four months before treatment. After treatment, his hands, fingers and wrists were completely normal except for a slight stiffness in one finger, which, they believe, will disappear with further treatment.

Here is a list of signs and symptoms that are usually found in people suffering from carpal tunnel syndrome. A feeling of "pins and needles" in hands, morning stiffness of fingers, impaired ability to flex the fingers; temporary paralysis of the arm and hand at night (they "go to sleep"), pain in hands and shoulders, pain on rotating the thumb, weakness of hand grip so that objects are easily dropped, night cramps in hands, feet or legs, pain or stiffness in knees, intermittent swelling of hands, impaired sensation in fingers (meaning that you cannot distinguish, from touching, a rough surface from a smooth surface), tenderness over the affected wrist, "pins and needles" in cheek or face, painful elbows, intermittent swelling of feet and ankles.

The authors of this very encouraging article discuss the possible reasons why only two milligrams of pyridoxine can apparently improve this painful condition slightly, while 100 milligrams of the B vitamin, continued daily for 11 weeks, can completely cure it. They do not know, now, they say, whether people suffering from this condition inherit a need for much larger amounts of the B vitamin than the rest of us, or whether they have for years just not eaten a diet which contains enough pyridoxine to sustain them in good health.

Why, then, do such people not show other symptoms of pyridoxine deficiency? Why is the deficiency manifested only in pain and stiffness? Some other symptoms of pyridoxine deficiency are: skin disorders, a kind of anemia, nerve problems that may lead to convulsions, and an increased excretion of a certain body compound. In animals, deficiency produces increased excretion of oxalates which may lead to kidney stones, also deficiency in insulin, the body hormone which controls the levels of blood sugar, increased excretion of urea, destruction of the myelin sheaths of the nerves (a condition which occurs in both polio and multiple sclerosis) and disorders of the adrenal glands.

The authors do not know, they say, why carpal tunnel syndrome should be the only indication of a pyridoxine deficiency in their patients.

"It may be," they say, "that there are diverse manifestations of vitamin B_6 deficiency, depending upon many variables and which have different degrees of occurrence in different individuals, including the presently recognized carpal tunnel syndrome."

So there is no way to be certain of results when or if you take increased amounts of pyridoxine to treat a painful stiff wrist with accompanying pain and stiffness in hands and fingers. But there seems to be no reason not to include this vitamin in goodly amounts in your daily supplements if you suffer from this condition, or even if your stiffness and pain afflict some other area of your body. Pyridoxine is harmless even in very large amounts, as are other members of the B complex of vitamins. You are perfectly safe in taking 100 milligrams or more daily. Don't expect overnight results. Vitamins are not drugs.

Dr. Ellis reminds us, too, that there almost has to be an association between carpal tunnel syndrome and diabetes, since it appears so often in those with diabetes or with diabetes in close relatives.

The important remedy for diabetes is, of course, changes in diet. And whether or not you have diabetes, the diet prescribed for diabetics is best for all of us, in any case, since it eliminates all refined carbohydrates from which all the fiber has been removed and concentrates on whole foods, natural foods with plenty of protein and plenty of fiber. This is the kind of diet we recommend always.

High protein foods such as lean meat, fish, poultry, eggs and dairy products are of paramount importance. Vegetables and fruits are essential—especially those with low carbohydrate content, like the leafy green vegetables and other salad "makings." All cereals and breads should be completely wholegrain which means getting them at the health food store or making them at home. They're just not available in supermarkets. Nuts and seeds are excellent sources of protein and fiber.

The B vitamins are of utmost importance to those who tend to have abnormal blood sugar levels—either too high, as in diabetes, or too low as in hypoglycemia. As we have seen, plenty of pyridoxine is essential for diabetics. It is removed almost completely when flour is processed to make white flour and it is never returned. It is removed completely when sugar cane is refined into white sugar and it is never returned. So it seems only reasonable that diets in which white flour, white sugar and highly processed cereals have been prominent would also be diets which promote diabetes and deficiency in the B vitamins, as well as vitamin E, many minerals and trace minerals.

We do not know if the actual biochemical process whereby the carpal tunnel syndrome is brought on will ever be fully explored and understood. But Dr. Ellis's work with individual patients demonstrates clearly the importance of pyridoxine in preventing and treating this painful condition. A good diet in which all refined carbohydrates are eliminated, is bound to help out, since it will provide much more pyridoxine, along with all those other nutrients which cooperate with it in the complex workings of body metabolism.

CHAPTER 13

Large Doses of Pyridoxine Used in Schizophrenia

TESTING URINE for the presence of a "mauve factor" has become a standard test for schizophrenia among physicians and psychiatrists who use megavitamin therapy in their treatment of this severe mental illness, which disables many thousands of Americans every year. Dr. Carl C. Pfeiffer explained why, in the December 14, 1973 issue of *Medical World News*.

Dr. Pfeiffer, who is now with the Brain Bio Center in Princeton, N.J., says that 30 to 40 percent of all schizophrenics excrete in their urine a certain substance which turns a deep pink or mauve when tested on a laboratory machine. As long ago as 1963, Dr. Abram Hoffer of Saskatoon and Dr. Humphry Osmond discovered this fact and published it in medical journals. Opponents of their theory said that the mauve color represented only a reaction to the tranquilizers being given to the schizophrenic patient. But the substance in urine has now been identified and is known to be something which the disordered, unbalanced body chemistry of the mentally ill person is excreting.

Dr. Pfeiffer tells of a patient who arrived at his clinic in 1971 suffering from "an unrelenting inferno of mental and bodily suffering." She had suffered over the years from insomnia, loss of reality, attempted suicide, seizures or convulsions, vomiting and difficulty with menstruation. She had been given nerve tests and psychiatric tests and they were normal. She had been hospitalized and tranquilized, all to no avail. Transferring from one hospital to another, she came at last to Dr. Pfeiffer who gave her chemical tests to determine her body's balance of nutrients—vitamins and minerals, and psychiatric tests to determine whether she suffered from perceptive disorders—that is, whether things looked peculiar to her, sounded peculiar, tasted wrong, smelled wrong.

He treated her with massive doses of pyridoxine and supplements of two trace minerals—zinc and manganese. He gave her group therapy and a tranquilizer. He believes, he said, that the food supplements should be given in two doses a day so that they flood the system of the patient.

This young patient improved with the vitamin-mineral therapy. When it was discontinued, she relapsed. Returned to this simple therapy she improved to such an extent that she has been free from convulsions for two years without other medication. She has made up the schooling she missed and is planning to become a doctor. Dr. Pfeiffer points out that she had trouble with knee joints when she began to menstruate. This gave him the clue that she might need two trace minerals, since lack of them produces similar troubles in animals.

The mauve chemical which is excreted in some schizophrenics seems to indicate that copper levels are normal in these people, whereas in other schizophrenics who do not have the "mauve factor" copper is lacking. The patient with "malvaria"—the mauve factor—may also have other symptoms: white spots on fingernails, loss of the ability to dream or to remember dreams after waking, a distinctive, sweetish odor on the breath and abdominal pain in the left side of the abdomen.

Other symptoms may be: constipation, inability to tan in sunlight, itching in sunlight, malformation of knee cartilages, joint pains. They may also have anemia, tremor and muscle spasms. They may be impotent or have menstrual difficulties, low blood sugar and an anemia which does not respond to iron but is improved when they are given pyridoxine.

Schizophrenics, doomed perhaps to a lifetime in mental hospitals, can benefit from this new knowledge of the physical, biological basis of their illness. And, says Dr. Pfeiffer, it's quite possible that, following this line of inquiry, we may discover many useful things about people who do not have the symptoms of schizophrenia.

Dr. Pfeiffer is one of the group of dedicated psychiatrists working with the Huxley Institute of Biosocial Research at 1114 First Avenue, New York City, 10021. If you know someone suffering from the terrible symptoms of schizophrenia, get in touch with the Institute and ask them for literature on this subject. They will be glad to direct you to psychiatrists in your locality, if there are any who are using nutritional therapy and megadoses of vitamins and minerals, along with more conventional therapy, to treat this disorder.

A paperback, *Megavitamin Therapy*, by Ruth Adams and Frank Murray, published by Larchmont Books, gives details about the therapy and many addresses of helpful, knowledgeable people. Ask for it at your health food store.

An innovative textbook for doctors is *Orthomolecular Psychiatry*, by Drs. David Hawkins and Linus Pauling, W. H. Freeman Co., 660 Market St., San Francisco, Calif., $17.00.

Getting back to zinc, it's a trace mineral which is being studied intensely these days because it has been found to be helpful in treating so many of our common disorders—acne, for instance. Now a U. S. Department of Agriculture biochemist has discovered that vitamin B_6 helps in the absorption of zinc. Dr. Gary W. Evans found that when rats were fed normal dietary levels of zinc they absorb one and one half times as much of it when they are given large doses of vitamin B_6 than when they are given smaller doses. Seventy-one percent of the zinc was absorbed when large doses of the vitamin were given whereas only 46 percent was absorbed when smaller doses were given. Dr. Evans was referring to really large doses of this vitamin—40 milligrams per kilogram. In a human being that would translate to about 3,000 milligrams for a 150-pound adult. The official dietary allowance for pyridoxine is 2 milligrams for an adult.

The trace mineral zinc has been used in large doses to treat acne, diabetes, wounds that will not heal, bone fractures, disorders of male sex organs, hardening of the arteries and many other disorders. Pyridoxine has been used to treat arthritis, carpal tunnel syndrome, convulsions, and many complications of pregnancy, including morning sickness.

The two nutrients occur in many of the same foods and many of these are foods from which practically all the pyridoxine and the zinc have been removed—the refined carbohydrates which include all sugar, white flour and all products made from it as well as processed supermarket cereals. By restoring these two valuable nutrients to your diet you can probably aid in the helpfulness of both, since the more pyridoxine you take, the more zinc will be absorbed.

Both nutrients are available in supplements. And it's a good idea to eliminate from meals and snacks all those foods from which zinc and pyridoxine have been removed—the refined carbohydrates. Replace them with real, wholegrains and fresh fruits rather than sugary desserts. Our information about zinc and pyridoxine comes from *Chemical and Engineering News* for November 5, 1979.

CHAPTER 14

Pyridoxine in Treatment of Convulsive Disorders

A CONVULSION is defined as an involuntary, uncontrollable seizure, involving muscular contractions. The history of pyridoxine is replete with case histories of individuals, infants and adults, who have suffered convulsions because of lack of this B vitamin. The only conclusion one can come to is that this B vitamin is extremely important for the health of brain, nerves and muscles, since all these are involved in convulsions.

Nutrition Reviews for January, 1975 contained a review of material on the subject in which the conclusion was stated that effects of vitamin B_6 on central nervous systems are not confined to that period in the life of an infant when the brain is developing. They are also associated with adults and with deficiencies of the following B vitamins; thiamine, riboflavin, niacin, folic acid and biotin.

Detrimental effects of pyridoxine deficiency on the central nervous system have been reported in both human beings and animals. In rats a deficiency in this B vitamin, while the young are still nursing and active brain development is in progress, can result in seizures and changes in electroencephalograms. Giving the B vitamin reversed the symptoms. In animals deficient in pyridoxine the brain protein is reduced, along with DNA and RNA which are cell elements that are essential for cell reproduction.

Says *Reviews*, "The recent studies . . . leave little doubt that the deficiency of many B complex vitamins in early or adult life can have profound effects on the central nervous system. The implications of such abnormalities in brain function on the overall performance of populations where widespread malnutrition exists need attention and investigation."

The January, 1976 issue of the same publication discusses vitamin B_6 deficiency in pregnant women.

"Biochemical assessment suggests that many pregnant women *consuming apparently adequate* diets may be in a poor state of vitamin B_6 nutriture," says *Reviews*. "In several pregnant women oral lesions considered to be due to riboflavin (B_2) deficiency were found to respond to pyridoxine."

The official recommended daily allowance for pregnant women is 2½ milligrams of pyridoxine, which does not seem to be enough, according to this article. Women who got 10 milligrams daily of the B vitamin had sustained, normal levels of pyridoxine throughout their pregnancy. And their infants were born in a good nutritional state where this B vitamin is concerned. Suggestions have been made that the recommended level be increased to 15 or 20 milligrams daily.

"The benefits which might be derived from these high levels, which obviously cannot be obtained from ordinary foods, are unknown but this is an area requiring continuing investigation," says *Reviews*.

One reason why increased amounts of this B vitamin may be necessary is that individual babies may have increased need for the vitamin. *The Journal of the American Medical Association* reported in February 7, 1966 on several infants who appeared to have greatly increased need for this vitamin.

One child born of an uncomplicated pregnancy died in convulsions within a day, although there was no history of nervous symptoms in his family. Another child had a history of convulsions which occurred every time she was taken off pyridoxine supplements. Such children have a "dependency" on pyridoxine, says the author, Dr. M. Moreno Robins of Provo, Utah. By this he means that they just naturally need far larger doses of this B vitamin than the rest of us need and they must have these large doses or they cannot survive. Their convulsions are not responsive to the usual drugs given to prevent convulsions, even when they are given in heavy doses.

Says Dr. Robins, "Treatment consists of 10 to 100 milligrams of pyridoxine hydrochloride administered intravenously or intramuscularly. The exact amount needed has not been determined and may actually vary somewhat in individual cases. Convulsions cease entirely within seconds after the parenteral administration of pyridoxine. If our case is typical, one dose will last three to six days before irritability, hyperreflexia, auditory stimuli, and finally convulsions recur. Daily maintenance therapy four to 10 milligrams administered orally is necessary to maintain the child symptom free. . . . Treatment may be required indefinitely. . . ."

A Czech medical journal reported in 1967 on intrauterine convulsions in three children born to the same mother. The first child died after seven weeks, the second the day after birth, the third survived. Convulsions in the uterus could be controlled by giving the mother pyridoxine. The Czech doctors recommend that pyridoxine "dependency" should be considered in families with abortions and still-births, especially if the pregnant woman reports fetal movements of a convulsive nature.

An article in *Nutrition Reviews*, March, 1967 described pyridoxine "dependency" in detail reminding its readers that the drugs commonly prescribed for epileptic convulsions are not effective in alleviating the ones caused by pyridoxine deficiency. But giving the B vitamin intravenously will stop the convulsions within minutes.

The state of dependency apparently is permanent, since discontinuation of pyridoxine supplements, even after years of treatment. . . ." results in a recurrence of convulsions 36 hours to five days later . . . The underlying defect in pyridoxine dependency seems to be an aberration in the metabolism of vitamin B$_6$ and not a simple dietary deficiency." Not getting enough of the B vitamin, however, appears to be so serious that permanent brain damage may result.

In 1974 Dr. David B. Coursin reported in *Family Practice News* that vitamin B$_6$ is of great value in treating schizophrenia, Down's Syndrome, myoclonic seizures and mental retardation. And, as we know from the work of many orthomolecular psychiatrists, pyridoxine is indeed very powerful in treating mental disorders of children, especially such conditions as autism, schizophrenia, hyperactivity and so on.

Adelle Davis, in her book *Let's Get Well*, recommends magnesium and pyridoxine for muscle and nerve disorders of many kinds including tics, twitching, muscle spasms, tremors. She also relates many documented stories of epileptic attacks which were overcome with pyridoxine, although she cautions that epilepsy which is not caused by lack of pyridoxine does not respond. It appears that quite a few cases do respond, indication that they *are* caused by lack of the vitamin or greatly increased need for the vitamin.

In most cases giving magnesium as well helps in the treatment. She says, "Muscle biopsies of babies who developed convulsions resulting from magnesium losses through diarrhea showed only half the normal magnesium content. These infants also had intermittent foot and wrist spasm, rigidity of the back and neck and tremors of the arms and legs, all of which became worse when water, given to overcome dehydration, diluted their magnesium supply. As soon as 500 milligrams of this nutrient were given them, all symptoms promptly disappeared. Because of a high calcium intake, infants are especially subject to a magnesium deficiency."

Almost 25 years ago, says Davis, Dr. Tom Spies, the distinguished physician who stopped the pellagra epidemic in our South, gave vitamin B_6 to people with epilepsy and got excellent results. Giving adequate magnesium as well as vitamin B_6 has achieved even better results with epilepsy patients. She tells us of 30 epileptic children who were given 450 milligrams of magnesium daily and could discontinue all drugs designed to control their attacks. Of the 30 children, only one child, who may have been deficient in vitamin B_6, did not show marked improvement on the magnesium treatment.

The two nutrients, magnesium and vitamin B_6, turn up again and again in nutritional literature, working together. Apparently this is a twosome which all of us should be aware of. Fortunately, they occur abundantly in the same groups of food so that attention to good diet can perhaps provide enough of each of them. However, as the story of pyridoxine shows so clearly, some individuals have greatly increased need for pyridoxine. When this need is such that they cannot live without these large amounts, we call it "dependency." And we must deal with it if the indivudal is to live a healthy life.

As we have reported several times in this book, individuals, especially babies, often require larger than usual amounts of vitamin B_6 because of a hereditary defect of certain enzymes for which the B vitamin serves as a coenzyme. In the affected babies, convulsions often result.

The Vitamin Information Bureau, Inc. tells us that one of the first demonstrations of B_6 deficiency purposely induced in humans took place in 1950. Dr. Selma Snyderman and her colleagues at New York University put two infants with congenital malformations on a diet in which pyridoxine was missing. One of the patients was a two-month-old child with hydrocephalus (water on the brain); the other was an eight-month-old child with microcephaly (abnormally small head).

"The infants failed to grow normally and showed biochemical signs of B_6 deficiency," the bureau reports. "B_6 in their urine diminished and when they were given a large amount of tryptophan (tryptophan load test) they excreted large amounts of xanthurenic acid, one of the breakdown products of tryptophan (this is regarded as an indirect sign of B_6 deficiency). The older child developed a progressively severe anemia which was corrected when one milligram a day of B_6 was added to the diet. The younger fared fairly well until the seventy-sixth day of B_6-free diet, when he suddenly had convulsions. This responded immediately to injection of 50 milligrams of B_6."

The bureau commented that the experiment showed two possible clinical reactions to pyridoxine deficiency in man: anemia and convulsions. However, the two conditions appeared unrelated, since the older child with anemia never had a severe seizure, even though he was not getting any pyridoxine for 120 days. Later, both conditions were discovered as independent syndromes, the bureau adds.

Soon after the New York experiment, during 1951-1953, spontaneous convulsive seizures of mysterious origin swept the country and doctors began to hunt for the cause of this epidemic of infantile epilepsy, continues the Vitamin Information Bureau, Inc. Doctors began describing a similar pattern that emerged in infants in all parts of the country: convulsions began suddenly in babies who previously had shown no signs of ill health. There were no other signs of illness and sedatives and anticonvulsant drugs were generally worthless. Some of the infants were only 18 weeks old.

"All were receiving the same synthetic liquid formula," the bureau comments. "On analysis, the formula was found to contain only 0.06 milligram of pyridoxine per liter, substantially less than the 0.1 milligram per liter content of human breast milk. Oddly, infants receiving the same formula in powdered form did not have convulsions. Apparently a considerable portion of B_6 in the formula had been destroyed in processing the liquid preparation."

Convulsions were prevented even if the babies were kept on the same liquid formula, providing that additional pyridoxine was given. The unwitting human experiment, the bureau notes, proved that without sufficient vitamin B_6 the brain is seriously affected. Since the babies were generally four months old or older before convulsions developed, it is assumed that they had sufficient tissue stores of the vitamin to tide them over, even though on an inadequate diet. After the B_6 in their bodies was depleted, the convulsions set in.

In 1954, the bureau reports, the Children's Hospital in Philadelphia, Pa., reported on a single case which turned out to be the prototype of a new syndrome—vitamin B_6 dependent seizures. The little boy had progressively severe seizures, which only responded to relatively high doses of pyridoxine. His diet contained sufficient B_6 for a normal child, but it was obviously not enough for him.

"There are now 17 known cases of this syndrome," the bureau says. "Convulsive seizures are common to B_6 dependency and B_6 deficiency states, but the onset is earlier in the former, the doses of B_6 needed to control the seizures are greater, and, if untreated or treated too late, the B_6-dependent child would very likely die in one of his fits. In fact, nine siblings of the 17 known cases have died in infancy under circumstances that strongly suggest that they had undetected B_6 dependency."

The bureau discusses one family in which two children died in convulsions and a third child was detected within the womb. From the seventh month of pregnancy, the woman became aware of convulsive movements of the fetus, the bureau continues. She was treated with 110 milligrams of B_6 a day, which stopped the fetal convulsions. The baby seems to have done well on 30 milligrams a day.

The bureau adds that convulsions are usually noted at birth

or within the first week after birth. However, in one child, the onset of the disorder was delayed until the third month. The amount of pyridoxine needed to stop the seizures has varied from two to 80 milligrams. Except in two cases, all of the children required a maintenance dose of vitamin B_6 far in excess of normal requirements.

"B_6 dependency is an inborn error of metabolism like PKU (phenylketonuria); galactosemia; maple syrup urine disease (an often fatal disease in which the infant's urine smells like maple syrup); and others that have received much attention lately," the bureau reports. "The exact nature of the underlying metabolic defect is not known, but the assumption is that the defect lies in some enzyme which requires B_6 as a co-enzyme. Perhaps a mutation has changed the structure of the enzyme so that it requires more co-enzyme molecules to function properly. At present the most likely suspect is glutamic acid decarboxylase, a B_6-requiring enzyme, that changes glutamic acid to gamma-aminobutyric acid (GABA). The latter is present mostly in the brain and appears to have an inhibitory effect on the nerve cells. A deficiency of GABA may directly or indirectly contribute to over-excitation and convulsions."

"Little did Hunt and his colleagues realize that they were witnessing a new phenomenon when they treated a 13-day-old infant suffering from constant and intractable convulsions which had begun three hours after birth," says an article prepared by Hoffman-LaRoche scientists.

"Pyridoxine deficiency was known at the time, but clinicians were not aware of any instance in which an abnormally high requirement for vitamin B_6 was associated with central nervous system disturbances," the article continues.

No drugs commonly used to control convulsions had any effect on this baby. But she remained free of the convulsions so long as the doctors continued to give her vitamin therapy. Finally they discovered that it was the pyridoxine in the vitamin pills that kept the convulsions at bay. And there seemed to be no way the infant could continue without this vitamin, for she developed convulsions whenever the therapy was discontinued.

"In the . . . years since Hunt termed a convulsive disorder 'pyridoxine dependency', much has been learned about inborn errors of metabolism, but many questions still remain unanswered. Pyridoxine dependency is described as a genetic disorder of newborn infants marked by generalized, massive seizures and subsequent mental retardation, if it is not treated early. Large doses of vitamin B_6 are required to control convulsions and to prevent structural changes which become irreversible. To remain seizure-free, the patient must be maintained on a quantity of pyridoxine in excess of the normal dietary intake, possibly throughout life."

We are familiar with the genetic condition called phenylketonuria in which newborn babies are unable to deal with one of the amino acids. They must immediately be placed on diets from which all this form of protein has been removed, or they will be mentally retarded.

At the time this article was written a number of years ago, only 25 cases of pyridoxine dependency had been reported in medical literature—far fewer than known cases of phenylketonuria. "But its clinical importance cannot be underestimated," say the scientists. "Despite its rarity, pyridoxine dependency is of great concern to the physician—particularly the obstetrician and pediatrician—because early recognition and treatment can prevent a disastrous clinical aftermath."

Urgent messages to other physicians have appeared in medical journals, alerting them to the dangers of convulsions in babies which can lead to severe mental retardation if they are not corrected at once. There are no ways to test individuals for pyridoxine dependence says the Hoffman-LaRoche article. So the physician must be ever alert always watching for visible signs and symptoms.

In cases of known dependency on pyridoxine there is usually a history of other infants in the family dying of convulsions soon after birth, although, in most cases, the reasons were unknown. This suggests that pyridoxine dependency is inherited.

Drugs which have been given in the past in attempts to stop the convulsions are: calcium gluconate, magnesium sulfate, intravenous and rectal paraldehyde and barbiturates (sedatives) and a drug used exclusively for convulsions. Not one of these elicited any response. But when pyridoxine was given the symptoms stopped dramatically—in one instance within a minute. The convulsions returned within 36 hours to 21 days and from then on it was necessary to give quite large doses of the vitamin to prevent further difficulties.

Note that the babies differed in their response to pyridoxine. It took 21 days for some of them to need more of the B vitamin while some needed it within three days. This says a great deal about our individual needs for this B vitamin. The need for early adequate treatment cannot be overemphasized, says the article. Of the 16 living children who are known to be pyridoxine dependent, only six are apparently normal. Three are mentally and physically retarded, one showed retarded development, one may have suffered permanent nerve damage.

The recommendations are that the individual be maintained possibly throughout life on doses of pyridoxine which may range from two milligrams up to three milligrams per pound of weight, which, in a 150 pound man, would be 450 milligrams daily. The experts who wrote this article also recommend that large doses of pyridoxine should be given to any mother who has previously given birth to a pyridoxine-dependent child. And to any mother who has a history of repeated stillbirth or who has a family background of unexplained death of newborns.

Since the cost is in pennies, there seems to be no reason

to ignore any of these recommendations. Taking large doses of pyridoxine is entirely without risk. Many people with no unusual symptoms of deficiency are taking them just to insure good health and to make certain that any extra personal needs are satisfied.

Other apparently inherited conditions in which pyridoxine deficiency is involved are these: Pyridoxine-responsive anemia, cystathioninuria, in which abnormally large amounts of an amino acid are excreted in urine. This, too, is associated with mental retardation and imperfect development of motor abilities. Familial xanthurenic aciduria is another inherited condition in which the processing of still another amino acid, tryptophan, is involved. In this condition too, far larger doses of pyridoxine than the average person needs are essential to keep the condition under control.

This is what we mean by "dependency." But it seems possible that this extreme need for very large doses of the vitamin in a few individuals may be important for all of us to remember. Perhaps many of us may have needs that are not this urgent or this life-threatening. But we may have inherited needs for much more pyridoxine (and other vitamins as well) than the average person.

CHAPTER 15

B Vitamins
for Treating
Autistic Children

SOME TIME AGO the following letter appeared in *The London* (England) *Observer*. Its author was Professor J. Noakes who teaches at an English university:

"Our child . . . was diagnosed as autistic by two different specialists at the age of two and a half and went into hospital for a year, though he came home at weekends.

"A biochemical test showed that he lacked pyridoxine (vitamin B_6). A number of other autistic children were tested at the same time and the same was found to be true of some of them though not of all. Since then we have been giving him the vitamin daily in pill form. About three months after we started, he said his first word (Bus!). Since then his improvement has been rapid and steady. He now has a vocabulary of approximately 400 words, he can use short sentences to express his wants and observations, understands the use of letters and numbers, and above all is beginning to appreciate other people. He will be five in December. His behavior is still autistic in many ways, but his progress judged by any standards, seems remarkable.

"At the time, our doctor was careful not to commit himself on there being a necessary connection between Oliver's improvement and the vitamin treatment, but he has published a preliminary report on his work in *Developmental Medicine and Child Neurology* for February, 1965. . . ."

In the massive volume entitled *Orthomolecular Psychiatry*, edited by David Hawkins and Linus Pauling, a chapter on treating mentally ill children with vitamins includes the above letter along with a great deal more information on the use of vitamins in larger than normal doses for children with behavior problems.

Says Dr. B. Rimland of the Institute for Child Behavior Research, San Diego, California, who wrote the chapter, "Because of articles appearing in the public press in the late 1960's concerning the controversy over Hoffer and Osmond's studies on vitamin use in adult schizophrenia, a number of the more adventuresome parents of schizophrenic and autistic children began experimenting with various combinations of the water-soluble vitamins to see if they could bring about some improvement in their children's condition. Many of these parents, aware of this Institute's role in serving as an information clearing house, began sending us reports of their experimentation and its results.

"Over a two-year period our initial skepticism was modified by the remarkably parallel reports trickling in from the parents and physicians of some twenty children in such widely separated places as California, New York, Massachusetts, Georgia, Washington, Canada and England."

Dr. Rimland and his associates sent a form letter to about 1,000 parents and doctors on their mailing list to locate additional children of high-dosage vitamin treatment. They got the case histories of 57 children and summaries from seven physicians who had used vitamins in treating children with severe behavior disorders.

Most of the parents had experimented on their own using

B vitamins in varying doses, sometimes as many as nine.

Says Dr. Rimland, "We were struck by the extent to which the trial and error efforts so often converged to the same group of three or four vitamins—the same vitamins that biochemical research studies have indicated as being of greatest relevance in mental disorder: niacin (vitamin B_3), ascorbic acid (vitamin C), pyridoxine (vitamin B_6) and, to a lesser extent, pantothenic acid (another B vitamin). Well over half the children for whom we received reports showed significant improvement, irrespective of diagnosis, and children given various combinations of these four vitamins in particular often showed remarkable improvement."

There was enormous diversity in the dosages of vitamins which these parents had decided upon. Niacin (or its other form niacinamide) was used in 40 of the 57 cases. It was given in levels ranging from 30 milligrams to 6 grams (6,000 milligrams) per day. Vitamin C, used in 27 cases, ranged from 100 milligrams to 6 grams per day. Doses of pyridoxine, which was used in 24 cases, ranged from 25 to 900 milligrams per day. Pantothenic acid which was used in 11 cases, was given in doses ranging from 25 to 900 milligrams per day.

In most cases dosage levels that appeared best were remarkably above the usual levels, although increasing them beyond the effective dose did not bring greater improvement.

Was it just a matter of "placebo effect," asked Dr. Rimland. Did the parents just believe in the treatment so firmly that they imagined their children improved? It's hard to say, says Dr. Rimland, since these were uncontrolled trials. But he points out that most of the children had such profound behavioral difficulties that improvement could not be missed, whereas children less drastically affected might, by chance, have good days and bad days.

The experimental use of massive doses of the water soluble vitamins took place in widely scattered communities, on a trial and error basis, yet the results show a clear consistency.

It was apparent that the best results were obtained when these vitamins were used consistently: niacinamide, pyridoxine and vitamin C. Most of these children had already been treated with a number of drugs with negative results or results that did not compare with the results of the vitamin therapy. After so many disappointments, says Dr. Rimland, one would expect parents to approach this new treatment negatively so that they would be inclined to discount anything that looked like improvement. Quite the contrary was true.

Several parents discontinued the vitamin treatment either because they wanted to see what would happen to the child, or because they just forgot to give the vitamins or ran out of them. They found that the child regressed suddenly and dramatically when the vitamins were discontinued and "there was often an equally dramatic improvement when the vitamins were reinstated," says Dr. Rimland.

"Although numbering perhaps only three or four per 10,000 among their peer group, children afflicted with the severe behavior disorders such as infantile autism and childhood schizophrenia, are victims of perhaps the most disabling illness known," says Dr. Rimland. Case histories of over 2,000 such children in the files of the Institute for Child Behavior Research show that psychotherapy and drugs are almost completely ineffective in treating these serious disorders.

Continuing his work with vitamin therapy, Dr. Rimland and colleagues, now at the Neuropsychiatric Institute of the University of California in San Francisco, reported in the *American Journal of Psychiatry*, April, 1978 on 16 autistic-type children who had improved when given just vitamin B_6.

He conducted a double-blind study of these children. That is, he gave the vitamin to half the group, giving a placebo (a "nothing" pill) to the other half. At the end of a specified time, the pills were reversed, with the first group getting the "nothing" pill, while the second group got the pyridoxine.

No one involved in the experiment, not the psychiatrists themselves, nor parents, nurses or the children ever knew which of these identical pills contained the B vitamin and which contained nothing but filler.

The behavior of the children was rated by the professionals and their parents while the children were being tested. Their behavior deteriorated "significantly" during the time the placebo was substituted for the pyridoxine which they had been receiving. And this in spite of the fact that no one knew whether they were still getting the vitamin, so there could be no psychological reason for either parents or doctors to expect these results.

The psychiatric establishment frowns officially on megavitamin therapy. One of their chief reasons is the scarcity of well-controlled double-blind tests like the one described here. The publication of this paper by Dr. Rimland in the *American Journal of Psychiatry* is a triumph over this official position. Perhaps individual psychiatrists may now be willing to at least try megavitamin therapy rather than drugs to see what success they may have.

The clue to success is the dose. Several milligrams of whatever B vitamin is involved—in this case, pyridoxine—will accomplish next to nothing. These badly damaged children need large amounts of B vitamins, especially niacin and pyridoxine, as Dr. Rimland has discovered.

We hope the day will soon arrive when all psychiatrists use diet and megavitamin therapy in treating the mentally ill, especially these children who are so seriously handicapped. The vitamins are completely harmless. They are obviously supplying the needs of young individuals whose needs are excessively high. We don't understand just why their needs are so high, but we don't need to understand that in order to use this therapy.

If you know of children who are suffering from autism or childhood schizophrenia, suggest that their families request information from the address below. This is a clearing house for information on the megavitamin-diet therapy for mental illness: Huxley Institute for Biosocial Research, 1114 First Avenue, New York, N. Y. 10021.

CHAPTER 16

Vitamin B₆ and Drugs

ONE MODERN ASPECT of nutrition which is almost totally ignored by the Nutritional Establishment as well as the Medical Establishment is at last getting the recognition it deserves through the publication of several books and many scientific papers on the subject of the nutritional harm that can be caused by drugs.

Modern drugs involve compounds of unimaginable complexity, each designed to treat some specific condition. The doctor can prescribe them with confidence, according to the drug company advertising. They will almost certainly relieve pain, correct glandular disorders, relieve stomach ulcers, lower blood pressure, prevent conception, cure skin disorders, and so on. Each individual drug has its purpose. But almost never does any drug advertising take up the subject of what the drug may be doing to the patient's nutritional state.

In a new book, *Drug-Induced Nutritional Deficiencies*, author Daphne A. Roe, M.D., tells us that drugs can interfere with the body's ability to manufacture certain nutrients. They can also affect the body's digestion and absorption of nutrients. And they can affect the way the body uses nutrients and excretes them. Drugs taken for short periods of time disrupt the nutritional state less seriously than drugs taken for a long time or for a lifetime.

In those of us who are obliged to take drugs for a long time, says Dr. Roe, the drugs, depending on their nature, will emphasize any pre-existing nutritional deficiencies caused by either not getting enough in meals or caused by disease. Since most diseases have some basis in nutritional deficiencies of various kinds, it seems apparent that drugs given for these diseases will probably make the existing nutritional deficiencies worse and may do so without anybody (including the doctor) being aware that this process is going on.

Pyridoxine appears to be one vitamin most seriously affected by a number of drugs in widespread use. Dr. Roe tells us that drugs which disturb the body's use of pyridoxine can produce nerve symptoms, including involvement of the central nervous system and convulsions. "In milder forms of B_6 depletion, depression is a common symptom," she says. (How many people do you know who are chronically depressed?)

Drugs which cause loss of pyridoxine in the body can bring on certain kinds of very serious anemia which can be life-threatening. They can also bring on symptoms of pellagra, that deficiency disease which usually involves the B vitamin niacin. When a drug is given that destroys pyridoxine, this can result in disordering the way the body uses the amino acid (protein) tryptophan and this can then cause loss of niacin which can produce the nerve, digestive and skin symptoms of pellagra.

Deficiency in either pyridoxine or the B vitamin folic acid can either produce or co-exist with deficiencies in other vitamins. Depletion of one vitamin affects the requirement for another. Both riboflavin (B_2) and niacin (B_3) stores in the body can be affected negatively when pyridoxine is lost.

Then there are the inherited conditions in which much

larger amounts of pyridoxine are needed by the person affected. There are five distinct genetic errors of metabolism which are dependent on pyridoxine, says Dr. Roe. In any of these cases the inherited condition must be identified by the physician and large enough amounts of the vitamin must be given throughout life. If the person is taking, at the same time, a drug which depletes the body of pyridoxine, the situation becomes even more serious.

"Levels of pyridoxine intake required by patients with pyridoxine-responsive diseases vary from 10 to 500 milligrams a day," says Dr. Roe. We're not talking here about small amounts.

Here are the names of some drugs which have been proven to disturb the body's use of pyridoxine, says Dr. Roe. The hydrazide drugs such as INH (given to lower blood pressure), and cycloserine which is an antibiotic derived from streptomycin. It is given for urinary infections and tuberculosis. According to *Drugs in Common Use*, "Convulsions have been reported following its use."

Convulsions appear over and over again in accounts of pyridoxine deficiency. Pyrazinamide and ethionamide (also given for tuberculosis) cause destruction of pyridoxine. Thiosemicarbizones (sorry, we could not find any material on what this drug is used for). Penicillamine (given to treat Wilson's Disease, an inherited disorder in which the trace mineral copper is stored in toxic amounts in the body.) L-dopa (Levadopa) used in the treatment of Parkinsons' Disease.

Among 50 patients who were given a drug in 1953 which induced pyridoxine deficiency, 34 developed the signs and symptoms of deficiency. The others did not. Among the symptoms were mouth and tongue disorders, conjunctivitis, seborrhea (a scaly skin condition), and later a severe nerve condition. Symptoms of pellagra appeared in some of the volunteers. All of these symptoms were relieved by giving pyridoxine in one form or another.

The two drugs mentioned earlier which are given for tuberculosis produce anemia in laboratory animals. Even when large amounts of iron were given along with the drug, the anemia was present, due to deficiency in pyridoxine. Some of these drugs, given alone, do not produce the characteristic anemia except in patients who have an inbred need for much larger amounts of the B vitamin. However if several such drugs are given at the same time the anemia is sure to result.

The hydrazine drugs given to lower blood pressure have the capacity to produce pyridoxine deficiency. This was reported as long ago as 1958. The nerve condition that was produced may have been caused both by the drug and by deficiency in the B vitamin before the drug was given.

One of the hydrazine drugs (monomethylhydrazine) produces not only deficiency in pyridoxine but also low blood sugar. So in order to prevent convulsions in laboratory animals to whom this drug is given not only pyridoxine but also intravenous glucose must be given, says Dr. Roe. No one knows if the same is true with human beings in regard to low blood sugar.

Another hydrazine drug used to treat cancer also produces deficiency in pyridoxine, along with serious nerve symptoms. Penicillamine is used in other conditions than the copper-storing disease. It is being used in disorders called macroglobulinemia and cystinuria. It has also been used in treating rheumatoid arthritis. And it has been advocated for treating patients with scleroderma, a skin and digestive tract disorder.

In 1966 a doctor used penicillamine in treating 13 patients with schizophrenia, our most serious mental disease. He knew that levels of copper are raised in the blood of these sufferers. He thought that this drug, which seizes on copper and causes it to be excreted, might help. Six of the 13 patients showed that they were developing deficiency in pyridoxine within four weeks of therapy. In another group of patients given the same drug, pyridoxine was also given and no signs of deficiency were observed. These doctors recommended that anyone taking D-penicillamine be given pyridoxine at the same time.

The history of several drugs given to treat tuberculosis is replete with many accounts of deficiency in pyridoxine produced by these drugs. Nervous symptoms were much the most common resulting in neuritis of various kinds. In some cases pellagra was also produced. Parasthesias, numbness, burning pain and weakness were produced in many patients, the severity of the condition depending on the amount of the drug that was given. The more drug, the worse the symptoms.

If the drug was discontinued, some symptoms might persist for as long as a year. The authors of one such report state that neuritis develops in *40 percent of all patients* on the drug isoniazid, usually within eight weeks of the beginning of treatment. Many investigators have testified to the beneficial effects of pyridoxine given at the same time as the drug. Fifty milligrams daily of the B vitamin were protective against nerve symptoms.

For a number of pages, Dr. Roe recounts experiments with human beings in which doctors studied the effects of this or that amount of the tuberculosis drugs. They measured various things in the patients' bodies to discover, if possible, just how much pyridoxine had been excreted, if any. They fussed over this or that aspect of the therapy, arguing over whether or not pyridoxine should be given in this or that circumstance.

The lay person reads this with impatience, wanting to force these nitpickers to give the B vitamin whether it may do any good or not! There's not a chance that it will do any harm. Why argue? Why nitpick? Why not give pyridoxine along with any drug you are giving, just in case the drug may be destructive of this B vitamin? Goodness knows, the drugs these doctors are giving are among the most expensive preparations in the world, while any B vitamin costs pennies, even when it is given in large amounts.

People who take drugs for tuberculosis and for high blood pressure are seen by their doctors frequently and may be checked for vitamin deficiencies, although the records do not indicate that all doctors or even most doctors look for such deficiencies. But what about the oral contraceptives which are one of the most commonly used drugs in the world today? What of the peasant woman in a South American or Asian country who gets her supply of The Pill once a year or so and doesn't see a doctor at all?

In a chapter on *Oral Contraceptives*, Dr. Roe discusses six vitamins and one trace mineral which are depleted in the bodies of many women when they are taking The Pill. One of these is pyridoxine. As long ago as 1966 a researcher showed that certain substances in the urine of women taking The Pill indicated pyridoxine deficiency. A number of other experiments on women taking The Pill demonstrated that depression apparently related to The Pill could be relieved by pyridoxine in some, but not all of these women. Presumably the doctors did not try larger doses of pyridoxine on those women who got no relief from the original dosage.

One study of 22 women with depression turned up 11 who had definite deficiency in pyridoxine. Giving the vitamin to these women relieved the depression, but had no effect on the other 11 women who showed no deficiency in the B vitamin. So we see that, as might be expected, some women are more likely than others to develop pyridoxine deficiency when taking The Pill. Every individual has different requirements for all vitamins. This should surprise no one surely. But is this any reason to withhold this totally harmless B vitamin from all women taking The Pill, since obviously not all of them will ever be tested for pyridoxine deficiency?

Why take a chance? Why not load that Pill with every vitamin and mineral known to be destroyed by the hormone in The Pill, just so that there is no chance for any woman to develop unexplained and unpleasant symptoms which may be due to plain deficiency in vitamins which is so easily treated.

We have a suspicion that the subject of drug-induced nutritional deficiencies is turning up just a few of the many many cases that will appear in the future as drugs become more complex and mysterious and their use more widespread.

Older folks these days take more prescription drugs than any other group in our nation. They are also most likely to be short on vitamins and minerals because of poor eating habits, and not enough money to afford highly nutritious foods. A one-a-day vitamin pill, selected on the basis of its composition in relation to the drugs being taken, along with supplemental tablets of pyridoxine and other vitamins which may be involved with these drugs seems not only wise but absolutely essential for the protection of these folks or anyone taking drugs for any length of time.

CHAPTER 17

"The Pill"
Destroys Vitamins,
Right and Left

FOR A NUMBER OF YEARS press releases have contained ominous statements in regard to oral contraceptives. First, the Food and Drug Administration gave official permission for the use of the "morning after" pill which is diethylstilbestrol, or DES. Two days earlier the head of the National Cancer Institute testified at a congressional hearing that women who take DES are likely to bear daughters who will later develop a rare and extremely serious vaginal cancer. Other people who testified at the hearings announced that the DES pill is already in widespread use among young women on campuses and elsewhere.

In February 1975 the American Medical Association printed in its *Journal* a somber article, prepared by a Group for the Study of Stroke in Young Women. This was a large group of professional specialists from universities and government bureaus. The conclusion they came to is that oral contraceptive use (that is, The Pill containing sex hormones) significantly increases the risk of disabling stroke in young women, even among those women who do not have high blood pressure. Either high blood pressure or cigarette smoking increases the risk of stroke.

On March 8, 1975 *The Lancet*, a British medical publication, published an article by a London physician in which he detailed the many vitamin deficiencies created in women who take The Pill. Vitamin A is increased in the blood of these women, for no reason that anybody understands as yet.

Of the B vitamins, riboflavin, pyridoxine, folic acid and vitamin B_{12} are deficient in women on The Pill. In other words something about the action which these powerful hormones have on the body depletes it of these essential vitamins. No one knows how or why, but it is a fact.

One would think, after the wealth of evidence this doctor presents that he would conclude his testimony by recommending that all women who insist upon taking The Pill be given vitamin supplements of these B vitamins, as well as vitamin C, for it has also been discovered that this vitamin is very deficient in women on oral contraceptives.

But no. After describing the life-threatening conditions produced by lack of these vitamins—especially the anemias related to folic acid and vitamin B_{12}—after describing the depression and disorders of blood sugar regulation produced by lack of pyridoxine, after noting that the condition of vitamin C deficiency produced is barely short of scurvy, this doctor says, well, we can't advise giving vitamin supplements because we just don't know what harm they might do!

He says this in spite of the fact that millions of people today are taking vitamin supplements daily, many of them are taking massive doses of the water soluble ones (B and C) and nobody has come to any harm. But faced with the real and terrible harm being threatened by The Pill, the physician feels that vitamin supplements are perhaps too dangerous!

The evidence on the way The Pill depletes vitamin stores has been piling up in medical journals year after year. As early as 1970 *The Lancet* published evidence that the depression of which many women on The Pill complain is caused by deficiency of vitamin B_6. Two Wisconsin physicians studied 58 patients who had been taking The Pill for an average of 14 months and who complained of at least three of these mental symptoms: emotional flareups and irritability, depression, fatigue, mild paranoia (they thought other people were persecuting them), difficulty with concentration and sleep disturbances.

Twenty-two of the patients had all five symptoms. Fifty had some of the symptoms before they started on The Pill, but the symptoms became worse on The Pill and new ones developed. The doctors gave them 50 milligrams of pyridoxine to take once daily when their premenstrual symptoms began. Eighteen reported complete cure of all symptoms. Twenty-six reported considerable improvement. Fourteen reported no change.

In those who noticed improvement with pyridoxine, the results were noticed within hours or by the next day at the latest. (This must have seemed like a miracle to women tormented with these troublesome symptoms.) The 14 patients who showed no improvement on 50 milligrams of pyridoxine daily were then given 100 milligrams—and still showed no improvement. No patients complained of any side effects.

One patient was so pleased with the results of the 50 milligrams of pyridoxine that she thought 100 milligrams would be even better. Every one of the 44 patients who improved on this vitamin therapy recommended pyridoxine to at least one friend or neightbor. One patient now has 12 friends taking the vitamin for mental symptoms.

Said these Wisconsin physicians, "These results support our clinical impression that pyridoxine is a valuable treatment for the five symptoms mentioned in patients taking oral contraceptives, and underlines the need for further research and controlled objective studies . . . the implications for treatment of premenstrual tension and pregnancy depression are obvious."

All 44 patients who improved were asked to discontinue pyridoxine to see if their symptoms returned. All refused to do so, because they were so pleased with the results. And even four patients who decided not to go on taking oral contraceptives because of their fear of side effects, went right on taking pyridoxine.

In November, 1970, another article appeared in *The Lancet* describing tests with 20 women using The Pill which showed that 16 of them had deficiency in vitamin B_6. The authors, from New York and New Jersey, point out that pregnant women experience a similar pyridoxine deficiency for several months only, but the long-term use of The Pill can result in a "chronic and sustained derangement in a large segment of an essentially young, healthy population. In view of its ready correctibility by oral pyridoxine," they ask, "might it not be advisable to recommend a vitamin B_6 supplement for users of The Pill?" Nobody answered their question, obviously, for few doctors seem to have noticed the pyridoxine deficiency produced by the pill they are giving.

In 1971 *The American Journal of Clinical Nutrition* printed an article by a group of New York physicians who studied 43 women all taking The Pill. They monitored the various changes brought about in the women as their supply of pyridoxine decreased. They point out in their article that various processes involved in the way The Pill acts in regard to pyridoxine can produce defective regulation of blood sugar levels and supply of insulin and can cause concern.

They tell us that the recommended daily allowance of two milligrams of pyridoxine given to the women corrected the deficiency in only 10 percent of them. The rest required 25 milligrams. Because they were studying so few women and it is well known (or should be well known by now) that different people may have widely different needs for various vitamins, they concluded that all women taking The Pill should be given 30 milligrams of vitamin B_6 daily along with The Pill. A totally harmless dose of a totally beneficial vitamin. But still no notice was taken of this suggestion by any official medical group or government health group.

In 1973 another *Lancet* article described the condition of 22 women on The Pill suffering from depression. This article states that about 80 percent of all women on The Pill are deficient in pyridoxine. About 20 percent have an *absolute* deficiency—no pyridoxine whatsoever in their bodies to perform the myriad processes for which this vitamin is responsible. Giving the women 20 milligrams of pyridoxine twice a day for eight weeks restored to normal the amount of pyridoxine their bodies needed.

The depression these women suffered included anxiety, dissatisfaction, lethargy, loss of sex drive, weepiness and irritability. The authors, from a London hospital, stated that it would be nice if they could recommend that every woman suffering from these preventable conditions should be given some pyridoxine to help her out, but, no. It might not work out, they say. No doctor protests the terrible toxicity of The Pill which is obviously destroying these women wholesale. But vitamin therapy to replace the vitamins The Pill has destroyed? No, that's too dangerous, according to these physicians.

Meanwhile, our extensive file on The Pill bulges with more and more medical articles relating newly discovered side effects of The Pill, all embellished with the quotation and disclaimer, "There is no such thing as absolute safety when it comes to contraception—you get nothing for nothing."

The Pill may be a cause of migraine headaches. The Pill may impair one's defense against infections. The Pill may bring vaginal discharges, urinary tract infections, susceptibility to chicken pox and other infections, eczema, loss of sex drive, mouth ulcers, high blood pressure, gall bladder troubles, serious alterations in results of laboratory tests which may throw off diagnoses of illness. Eighteen and a half million women were taking The Pill in 1969, undoubtedly many more than that by now. Periodically some researcher gives out a press release on research on the Male Pill but it's never any more than a press release.

And on March 5, 1975 the *New York Times* said that the development of safer methods of contraception is being seriously hampered because the multi-billion-dollar drug industry does not see any chance of making a pile of money out of a new pill before 1990 and that's too long to wait!

So go ahead and suffer, ladies. But don't take another milligram of pyridoxine or vitamin B_{12} or folic acid or riboflavin because nobody knows what they might do to you, says official medical authority. And it says this in spite of the fact that its own publications are bulging with evidence of the complete harmlessness of all these vitamins taken in massive doses over many years, along with massive doses of vitamin C. The drug companies just can't make any money selling vitamins, so it's up to young women to go right on suffering the evil effects of the vitamin deficiencies the profitable drugs (like The Pill) produce in a large proportion of all young American women. Such an attitude is scandalous and must be fought.

Pyridoxine is present most abundantly in those foods which contain the most of all the other B vitamins as well—wholegrain cereals, nuts, seeds, meat, poultry, fish, eggs, dairy products, fresh fruits and vegetables. It is also available at your health food store in inexpensive harmless vitamin supplements as are all the other B vitamins, and vitamin C.

CHAPTER 18

Kidney Stones, Bladder Stones and Vitamin B$_6$

KIDNEY STONES and bladder stones made up chiefly of calcium oxalate or a mixture of calcium oxalate and calcium phosphate "present a stubborn and curious puzzle to the urologist," says a review in the January, 1976 issue of *Nutrition Reviews*. There just doesn't seem to be much reason why certain individuals should suffer from these painful disorders, since they appear to be otherwise healthy and the amount of calcium in their blood appears to be "normal."

Symptoms of both kinds of stones are: pain and frequent, bloody urination. Small stones may pass out through the ureter. Larger stones which may block the flow of urine must be removed by surgery or some other method. Up to now, specialists have generally believed that bladder stones are caused by chronic inflammation of the bladder, enlargement of the male prostate gland, contraction of the neck of the bladder, a diverticulum or pouch in the wall of the bladder or kidney stones which have moved down into the bladder.

Now we are told in *Nutrition Reviews* that stones may be caused by deficiency in an important mineral and an equally important vitamin. The mineral is magnesium. The vitamin is vitamin B_6. A lengthy experiment involving some 150 people seems to show great improvement in the tendency to form such stones when people who are susceptible are given the two nutrients over a long period of time.

The experiment was accomplished by getting the aid of a large number of urologists who agreed to give the two nutrients to a given number of patients who could be expected to form a given number of stones in the time of the experiment—five years. About 150 patients were involved. Certain qualifications were set. Only patients who had formed at least one stone in the previous five years were accepted. They must also be free from urinary infection, have normal kidney function, normal levels of calcium and phosphorus in the blood and be free from other diseases which sometimes accompany stone formation—peptic ulcer, for example.

The volunteers were given a magnesium supplement consisting of 100 milligrams three times a day. By this we assume they took the tablets with meals. They were also given 10 milligrams of the B vitamin daily. No other change was made in diet or treatment.

The reduction in stone formation was dramatic. The group as a whole had formed an average of 1.3 stones before they began treatment. Taking the food supplements for five years resulted in an average of only one-tenth of a stone during the five years the test continued. Furthermore, *the only stones formed were limited to 17 of the 150 subjects*. The others had no stones at all during this five-year period. None of them suffered any side effects.

The *Nutrition Reviews* writer professes amazement at these results. What could they mean? he asks. Is it possible that the person who regularly forms kidney or bladder stones has a marginal deficiency in magnesium and/or pyridoxine either because he doesn't get enough at mealtime or because he just happens to need more than the average person? We would say, gentlemen, that both of these circumstances may certainly be the reason for formation of stones. Magnesium and pyridoxine are both found most abundantly in wholegrain cereals and breads as well as other seed foods. When white flour is made, most of the magnesium and pyridoxine are discarded and never replaced in the flour. Why should not modern human beings be short on both nutrients?

But, says the *Reviews* writer, these people did not seem to be suffering from a magnesium deficiency. And, what is more, people who are known to be suffering from a magnesium deficiency, as a result of lack of absorption, prolonged diarrhea, excessive alcohol intake or protein malnutrition, do not generally form stones.

In the case of pyridoxine, there seems to be even less evidence of a deficiency. In fact, it seems that the pyridoxine may not be necessary to the success of such a trial. An earlier experiment showed that magnesium supplements alone stopped the formation of stones in the people tested.

The article goes on to tell us that in laboratory rats on a diet low in magnesium bladder stones are *always* found. Calcium oxalate stones are *always* found in laboratory rats on a diet low in pyridoxine. In some experiments, where animals have been deprived of magnesium, a strongly alkaline urine and a reduced excretion of magnesium produced stones.

A diet low in magnesium, but high in phosphorus and moderate in calcium tends to cause stone formation in kidneys and heart. This kind of diet is probably widespread in our country, for meat is high in phosphorus, which tends to overbalance the lack of magnesium (found mostly in cereal foods and bread). When all the breads and cereals you eat have had their magnesium removed, the balance between the two minerals would be thrown out of kilter.

The question of why some otherwise healthy people tend to form stones while others do not, and why the addition of magnesium and pyridoxine should stop the stone formation remains a mystery, says *Nutrition Reviews*. But there is valuable evidence that this is so. Since the therapy is completely harmless this study "should encourage its wider application," says the magazine.

Nutrition Reviews is published by the Nutrition Foundation, a trade organization of the giant food industry. It is the official position of this industry that the American food supply is totally adequate in all respects and that it is totally impossible for any American eating "the average American diet" to be deficient in any nutrient. So one would expect that their publication would be unable to explain how two simple, essential nutrients, given in rather large amounts, might correct a long-standing disorder as serious as stone formation.

However we "food faddists" have known for years that many of us may be deficient in many nutrients, both because we cannot get enough of them at our daily meals and because we, as individuals, may have needs for individual nutrients far higher than "the average."

In a recent book, *Vitamin B₆, The Doctor's Report*, written by Dr. John M. Ellis, the relationship of magnesium and pyridoxine is clearly shown. Dr. Ellis relates stories of his patients who suffered from a variety of disorders which yielded to magnesium and pyridoxine supplements.

One is perfectly safe in taking far more pyridoxine than the 10 milligrams these doctors gave their patients. Many specialists are now requesting that this B vitamin be included regularly in all contraceptive pills, since it appears that women taking these pills are bound to be short on pyridoxine. Many other conditions of ill health are seemingly related to shortage of pyridoxine, due largely, one must believe, to its almost total absence from those foods which make up half the meals of many people—white sugar and white flour and everything made from them.

The table on page 129 shows the foods in which magnesium is most abundant. They are, generally speaking, the same foods in which the B vitamin pyridoxine is most abundant as well. See that your family gets enough of these foods every day. If there is any doubt in your mind, get magnesium supplements for your family. The recommended daily allowance of magnesium for adults is 300 to 400 milligrams. Children need less.

A French scientist, reporting in a recent issue of the *International Journal for Vitamin and Nutrition Research*, 44 (3), 1974, pp.344-46, fed one group of rats a complete highly nutritious diet, then gave two other groups diets deficient in pyridoxine, or deficient in magnesium or deficient in phosphorus. He found that getting not enough magnesium or enough pyridoxine interfered with the rats' growth. Not enough magnesium brought on skin troubles and gray hair!

Deficiency in both pyridoxine and magnesium caused retention of calcium and phosphorus in the kidneys and the pyridoxine-deficient animals excreted oxalate in the urine—which might easily lead to bladder or kidney stones. Whole grains, seeds and nuts are the best sources of phosphorus, pyridoxine and magnesium. Human diets which include plenty of such unrefined, unprocessed foods contain far more of these minerals than diets in which bread and pastries are made from white flour and cereals are the processed, supermarket kind.

Now if magnesium is involved with the health of skin and hair in laboratory animals, chances are that it's also important to the health of these parts of human beings.

If lack of both magnesium and pyridoxine can bring on retention of calcium in the kidneys, then this might very well explain the veritable epidemic of kidney stones and kidney troubles of many kinds which plague our nation today.

Dr. Abram Hoffer reminds us in the October, 1975 issue of the *Huxley Institute—SCF Newsletter* that pyridoxine is involved in the body's conversion of oxalate to glycine, the next step in metabolizing it. Oxalic acid is the substance in some foods which renders calcium unavailable to the body. That is, if you were to eat nothing but spinach, let's say, you might become quite deficient in calcium because spinach contains considerable oxalic acid.

But we don't eat diets consisting of nothing but foods rich in oxalic acid. We eat a variety of foods. And pyridoxine is in many foods, in any well planned diet. So we suffer no harm from the oxalic acid in spinach or the other vegetables that contain it. Is there a possibility of kidney stones from taking large doses of vitamin C? As you can see from the information above, it's lack of pyridoxine and/or the mineral magnesium which brings on kidney stones—not too much vitamin C.

Pyridoxine is a part of the body's processing material for fats, carbohydrates and protein. It participates in the enzyme activity which allows us to assimilate these food elements. So we could not conceivably get along without it. It is especially important in relation to the amino acid tryptophan. In diets where vitamin B_3 (niacin) is lacking, an amino acid, tryptophan, is converted into niacin in the body to prevent the vitamin deficiency disease of pellagra. This operation can take place only when there is enough pyridoxine present. So this is another important function of this vitamin.

It participates, too, in manufacturing certain body hormones such as histamine and adrenalin. Adrenalin is the hormone which is called up when you are under stress and need all the energy you can summon. So getting enough pyridoxine will help in this emergency. Pyridoxine is also important for the body's manufacture of certain blood elements which prevent anemia. So you must have it, if you would be safe from that debilitating disease.

Says Dr. Hoffer, "Since there is no definite vitamin B_6 deficiency disease as there is for vitamin C (scurvy), phy-

Milligrams of Magnesium in Four Ounces of Foods
(One Serving)

Almonds	270
Apricots, raw	62
Asparagus	20
Banana	33
Barley, whole grain	124
Beans, lima	67
Beets	25
Beet greens	106
Brazil nuts	225
Cashew nuts	267
Chard, Swiss	65
Corn, fresh	147
Cottonseed flour	650
Cowpeas (Blackeyed peas)	55
Dandelion greens	36
Filberts	184
Lentils	80
Millet	162
Oatmeal, wholegrain	169
Peanuts	206
Peanut butter (1/3 cup)	82
Peanut flour	360
Peas	35
Pecans	142
Pistachios	158
Rice, brown	88
Rye flour (whole)	73
Sesame seeds	181
Soybeans	265
Soybean flour, defatted	310
Walnuts	190
Wheat bran	490
Wheat germ	336
Whey, dried	130
Yeast, brewers	231

sicians have not been trained to look for evidence of pyridoxine deficiency. The daily B_6 intake recommending up to two milligrams per day has no meaning since it ignores wide-ranging differences between people. The need varies with the state of health, with the amount of protein consumed (more protein consumed requires more vitamin B_6). Many scientists are worried about the adequacy of our food with respect to B_6."

He then quotes a noted nutrition expert, Dr. Nevin Scrimshaw, who said in 1967, "Early malnutrition which stunts growth has also clearly and repeatedly been shown in experimental animals to reduce subsequent learning ability, memory and behavior. To the extent this is true for young children as well, the generations on whom social and economic progress will depend in the remainder of this century are being maimed now in body frame, in nervous systems and in mind."

So a deficiency in vitamin B_6 can bring on the following effects:

1. Convulsions in babies.

2. You can get painful neuritis from lack of pyridoxine. A number of drugs destroy the vitamin (isoniazid, penicillamine, etc.).

3. You can get anemia from lack of pyridoxine.

4. You can get kidney stones.

Dr. Hoffer tells us of experiments in which animals made deficient in pyridoxine were given magnesium and the expected kidney stones did not materialize. "Out of 36 (human) patients who were chronic oxalate stone formers, 200 milligrams of magnesium oxide and 10 milligrams per day of vitamin B_6 over five years prevented recurrence or greatly decreased it in 30."

There are people who need far more pyridoxine than the rest of us. Dr. Hoffer believes that as many as five percent of any "normal" population and up to 75 percent of a severely ill psychiatric population have this problem. They need more pyridoxine than they can get in the average diet.

"As well as being mentally ill," he says, "these patients may have constipation and abdominal pains, unexplained fever and chills, morning nausea, especially if pregnant, hypoglycemia (low blood sugar), impotence or lack of menstruation, and neurological symptoms such as amnesia, tremor, spasms and seizures. The treatment consists of optimum amounts of B_6 and zinc." About one-third of all schizophrenics suffer from this need for very large amounts of the vitamin. And, as we have said, there is much evidence that The Pill, the oral contraceptive, is destructive of pyridoxine.

We are told that the amount of fat in American diets has a lot to do with our soaring figures on heart disease and deaths from heart attacks. Since pyridoxine is one of the vitamins involved with processing fats in the body, might it help to prevent heart troubles? It seems so. Scientists have shown that monkeys getting high-fat, high-cholesterol diets do not get artery troubles if they are getting as much as five milligrams of pyridoxine a day. This means that human beings should be getting about 25 milligrams daily if they want the same protection. But here again, we have individual needs which may be higher.

If you eat a really well-planned diet you are getting considerable pyridoxine. Best sources are: all kinds of liver, herring, salmon, walnuts, peanuts, wheat germ, bran, brown rice, brewers yeast and blackstrap molasses. Medium good sources are meat, especially organ meats like kidney and heart, fish, eggs, wholegrains, legumes (peas, beans, soybeans, lentils) and leafy green vegetables like kale, brussels sprouts, spinach and so on.

Keep in mind that you cannot depend on bakery bread as a source of pyridoxine. This is one of the B vitamins which disappears when white flour is made. It is never returned in the "enrichment" program. So it is missing from white flour.

Most commercial bread is made largely from white flour (even the wholegrain and pumpernickel kinds) so you will get almost no pyridoxine from such bread. Make your own bread from real wholegrains available at the health food store or buy real wholegrain bread which is sold there.

Wheat germ and bran are other excellent sources which you should use to enrich every food you prepare for the table. Add them while you are cooking. Drop some into the white sauce, the soup, the meatloaf. Sprinkle them on top of whatever cereal you are eating, stir them into the oatmeal. At all costs, make certain you are getting enough pyridoxine, for the sake of your nerves, your heart, your digestion, your skin.

CHAPTER 19

This Orthomolecular Psychiatrist Takes Lots of Pyridoxine

ABRAM HOFFER, M.D., President of the Huxley Institute for Biosocial Research in New York, believes that senility (those mental problems that beset many older folks) is a form of chronic malnutrition. He takes large doses of certain vitamins and minerals in an effort to prevent senility in himself. Here are his comments on this subject at the National Conference sponsored by the Huxley Institute in 1972.

I want to talk briefly about an experiment of nature that was made involuntarily.

In 1940 the Japanese captured 2,000 Canadian soldiers defending Hong Kong. They were in prisoner-of-war camps for 44 months—nearly four years. Most of the men who survived had lost a third of their weight, and had suffered from many infections and from pellagra, beriberi and just about every other deficiency disease known. The survivors were admitted to hospitals in Canada, where they received what was then considered massive doses of vitamins—for example, 50 milligrams a day of nicotinic acid (a form of vitamin B_3 or niacin.)

These veterans have since then been a perpetual problem. They are complaintive, neurotic, never seem to do well. One of these veterans is a long-time close friend of mine. In 1960 he was typical of these veterans—chronically complaining, neurotic, depressed, fatigued, with arthritis and neuritis. Every morning it took the combined efforts of his wife and himself to get him out of bed so he could be mobile.

At that time, after talking with me about some nicotinic acid research I was proposing, and after being reassured that I did not think it was dangerous, he started taking three grams a day—30 times as much as before. (Three grams is 3,000 milligrams.)

In only two weeks this man had recovered, and he has remained well since then—except for a short period in 1962 when he went mountain climbing in the Rockies—at the age of 58—and forgot his vitamins.

Within two weeks his joints started freezing, his arthritis was returning, he was again becoming very depressed and tense. He has never made this mistake again, and remains well to this day.

Now this one case doesn't prove anything, but it is certainly a dramatic picture of the effect of nicotinic acid on one man.

The other Hong Kong veterans received large quantities of amphetamines by day and barbiturates in the evening until tranquilizers arrived and replaced the barbiturates.

A study released in 1965 showed that all but 12 had many of the signs and symptoms of aging, often in extreme degree—with apathy, fatigue, insomnia, anxiety, irritability, depression, peptic ulcer, irritable bowel, atherosclerosis (hardening of the arteries), a 70 percent higher coronary death rate than a control group of Canadians who had been in European prisoner camps, poor dental health, optic atrophy (they seemed to be going blind at a rapid rate).

The dozen exceptions had started taking truly massive quantities of nicotinic acid 10 years ago, and—as far as we can tell—are now normal.

Well, this means we may be dealing with a new category of deficiency disease that I would like to call acquired dependency disease. There is a new class of diseases called dependency disease. Apparently we know of about 13. By definition, a dependency disease is the condition in which the patient requires substantially larger quantities of a particular vitamin than the average person, even on the order of perhaps a thousand times as much.

Many years ago, it was shown that if you produced black tongue or pellagra in animals by depriving them of vitamin B_3 for a month or so, you could reverse this effect by giving them the usual dosage of nicotinic acid (B_3) related to their size. But if you prolonged the B_3 deficiency up to six months, the animal no longer responded to the usual dosage and required megadoses (very large doses) of nicotinic acid to restore and maintain his health.

It was also known that in chronic pellagra it might take a daily maintenance dose of up to 600 milligrams a day of nicotinic acid just to keep the patient from becoming psychotic.

So it seems that when people are long deprived of nutritional supplements, especially vitamins, they may acquire a dependency disease. I think that senility is, in fact, merely a chronic form of malnutrition.

In orthomolecular medicine, our approach is based on Dr. Roger Williams' work stressing biochemical individuality, and on Dr. Linus Pauling's work, starting with his famous 1968 paper in *Science* on "Orthomolecular Psychiatry." Pauling's thesis was simply that you must provide the optimum quantity of nutrients in the right organ at the right time.

So, to stave off senility, we have to take the following

factors into account:

1. Adequate diet, with appropriate vitamins and other supplements properly balanced.

2. Adequate absorption into the blood stream.

3. Adequate circulation through the body.

4. Adequate utilization with presence of necessary hormones and coenzymes.

5. Accelerated detoxification, to get rid of clinkers.

I try to reflect all these things in my prescriptions for my own patients who are becoming senile. In addition, let us all stop smoking. Dr. Pauling has shown that the average person who smokes one pack a day shortens his life by eight years. Two packs, 16 years. There's your choice.

Let us cut down on radiation exposure. Let us reduce the content of toxic matter, especially in the air we breathe. Let us be more concerned with detoxifying mechanisms. Some of us are now doing research on fasting therapies. Fasting might be a nice way to help the body get rid of the toxins we have ingested. I repeat that I believe senility is a form of chronic malnutrition.

I am now running an experiment on myself. If I survive to 90, I will have some data. I am taking at least 30 vitamin pills a day—including four grams of nicotinic acid; 4 grams of ascorbic acid (vitamin C); 800 units of vitamin E; 250 milligrams of thiamine; 250 milligrams of pyridoxine; vitamins A and D; some calcium, iron and a mineral supplement. I now feel fine, but later I may not. I'll let you know in 40 years.

CHAPTER 20

Trying to Have a Baby? Vitamin B₆ May Help

SOME OF THE 14 women had been trying unsuccessfully to conceive for seven years, others for 18 months. Twelve of the women became pregnant after they were given a course of treatment with large doses of vitamin B_6, also known as pyridoxine.

Their doctors do not know why the treatment was successful, says *Medical World News* for March 19, 1979. They think the vitamin may suppress a certain hormone called prolactin which is concerned with lactation and certain other aspects of pregnancy.

Five of the women studied showed no evidence of suppression of this hormone by the vitamin, so the answer must lie elsewhere. In any case, 13 pregnancies resulted from the vitamin treatment (one woman conceived twice). Of the two women who did not become pregnant, one dropped out after adopting a child, the other after a divorce.

The vitamin was given in doses ranging from 100 milligrams daily to 800 milligrams daily for at least six months or until conception occurred. Eleven of the pregnancies occurred in the first six months, one in the seventh and one in the 11th.

Director of Reproductive Endocrinology at Duke University, Dr. Charles B. Hammond, called the results "intriguing" and urged more investigations in a double-blind controlled trial. In such a trial half of the women involved would be given a "nothing" pill while the others took the vitamin, to see if only those taking the vitamin would become pregnant.

This approach is the usual medical approach. Doctors continue to believe that vitamins are just the same thing as drugs and must be treated as "miracle" potions which produce results almost at once. This is not the way things work. Vitamins are food. If indeed, large doses of pyridoxine produce pregnancy in hitherto infertile women, this doesn't mean that this vitamin is a miracle drug. It means that these infertile women have not been getting enough pyridoxine in their meals up to now, or it means that their needs are far greater than "average." The large doses given are simply supplying the amount of the vitamin necessary to make these women "normal," hence able to conceive.

It is not the least surprising that large numbers of American women should lack vitamin B_6. It is removed almost entirely from all those foods which make up half the average American diet—the refined carbohydrates, white flour and white sugar chiefly. It is never replaced in any of these foods, although three other B vitamins are replaced in an "enrichment program."

So a diet that lacks pyridoxine produces defective operation of all those body functions that depend on this vitamin. It is needed for processing protein, carbohydrate and fat in the body. It is essential for almost anything that involves the use of protein by the body. It helps the liver to produce blood sugar from protein. It is used in the production of hormones that control nerves. The body needs it to produce essential unsaturated fatty acids. It is needed to prevent certain kinds of anemia.

Perhaps most important to a consideration of infertility is the fact that pyridoxine is destroyed wholesale by The Pill, the oral contraceptive. We are not told whether the women involved in this experiment had been taking The Pill. If they were and if they had been eating the average American diet, (woefully short on pyridoxine) then their deficiency would be excessive, so all those functions for which this B vitamin is needed would be bound to suffer.

Of course, large amounts of the vitamin would be necessary to correct such a deficiency. And perhaps some of the women had inherited much higher needs for this vitamin than the rest of us have. The account of this triumph over infertility does not describe any ill effects from the large doses of this vitamin. Of course there were none. The vitamin has been given in much larger doses than these without any uncomfortable side effects. All the B vitamins are water soluble, so any excess is excreted harmlessly within a few days.

None of this has much to do with having a baby, you may say. But it does indicate how intricately this vitamin is woven into almost everything our bodies do. So to say there is no obvious "deficiency" disease caused by lack of pyridoxine is a half truth. Perhaps epilepsy or other convulsive diseases are diseases of pyridoxine lack. Perhaps all or most abnormal accumulations of minerals causing stones in various parts of the body are indications of pyridoxine deficiency. Perhaps neuritis, anemia, mental illness are indications of pyridoxine deficiency, along with other deficiencies which are quite likely to accompany deficiency in vitamin B_6.

Perhaps infertility is chiefly a disorder of pyridoxine deficiency.

CHAPTER 21

Vitamin B₆ Is Essential in Pregnancy

"ALL PREGNANT WOMEN have an increased need for vitamin B_6," says Dr. John Ellis in his book *Vitamin B_6, the Doctor's Report*. He tells us that during pregnancy many common symptoms appear which can be treated with pyridoxine (vitamin B_6). Some of these are swollen hands and feet, leg cramps, hands and arms that "go to sleep," and other nervous symptoms in hands and arms.

But most of all, he says, vitamin B_6 plays an important part in preventing and treating toxemia of pregnancy and the convulsions that occur in eclampsia, the dreaded disease of late pregnancy. Eclampsia involves high blood pressure, edema, protein in the urine, and convulsions or coma.

Dr. Ellis says that edema (unnatural accumulation of water in tissues resulting in swelling) is present in at least one-third of all pregnant women in our country. It may lead to eclampsia which is a life and death situation for both mother and child.

"It is accepted by now that proper nutrition is more important during pregnancy than at any other time," says Dr. Ellis. "For this reason, any woman who suspects that she may be pregnant should check with her physician immediately so that he can advise her on her nutritional obligations to herself and her unborn child. He will insure that she is instructed as to a balanced diet that contains sufficient minerals and vitamins as she 'eats for two', and he will prescribe vitamin-mineral supplements . . . sufficient vitamin B_6 supplements will play an essential role during the nine months following conception."

Unfortunately all physicians are not as knowledgeable about nutrition as Dr. Ellis is. During the past 10 years or so many obstetricians all over the country have been obsessed with preventing their patients from gaining weight and have, in many cases, put them on diets that were low in calories but shockingly deficient in essential nutrients. Fearing edema, they have also forbidden the use of salt and any foods that contain it. And, in most cases, have given these pregnant women powerful diuretics (water pills) that have brought about the loss of still more essential nutrients.

Most young people today were brought up on diets high in salt. To switch suddenly to low salt diets has made food for many pregnant women so unappetizing that they simply don't eat enough to sustain good health for themselves and the baby. Medical journals continually point out that doctors know almost nothing about nutrition, since they have almost no training in it, so how could they manage to design a perfectly nourishing diet for a pregnant woman who has to shop at a supermarket with the many traps for the unwary that crowd the shelves?

Laboratory evidence as to the increased need for B_6 during pregnancy is well established, says Dr. Ellis. Dr. Paul Gyorgy, a distinguished expert in the field of B vitamins, has said that all pregnant women studied have shown, by laboratory evidence, that additional B_6 is necessary to normalize the excretion of certain compounds in the urine. Any woman who has been pregnant will agree, says Dr. Ellis, that this condition makes more major changes in the human body than any other circumstance.

Dr. Ellis tells us of 225 pregnant women in his care who were treated successfully *without* salt restriction and *without* the use of diuretics. He used vitamin-mineral supplements or supplements of B_6 alone. In the beginning, fearful that he might give overdoses of the B vitamin, he used available prenatal capsules which contained from 3 to 10 milligrams of B_6. Ten milligrams seemed to be enough for many of his patients. But others seemed to need far more to treat many symptoms—like the following.

Many of his patients described numb arms when they awakened in the morning. One arm would appear to be almost paralyzed, so that they had to use the other hand to massage it. This one symptom came to indicate clearly the need for additional B_6, says Dr. Ellis. Leg cramps, "pins and needles" in hands and arms, and painful finger joints also responded to B_6, but the amounts needed varied greatly. Some of his pregnant patients needed as much as 450 milligrams of pyridoxine before they overcame the pain in finger joints.

Leg cramps are a frequent complaint of pregnant women, he says. They are usually ascribed to deficiency in calcium. But, he says, he has seen painful leg cramps in women on high calcium diets. Usually plenty of pyridoxine relieved the cramps. When it didn't he sometimes gave potassium supplements. And later he discovered that magnesium supplements were very good for stopping the cramps.

He describes one case of a woman of 39 in her eighth pregnancy. Her mother was a diabetic. On one occasion the pregnant woman's urine showed traces of sugar. She had painful fingers and legs, edema in feet and legs and severe muscle spasms in her legs at night. Fifty milligrams of pyridoxine daily, in addition to the 10 milligrams in her vitamin-mineral capsule, obliterated the cramps. She lost eleven pounds, obviously fluid, and the edema disappeared almost entirely. Although her blood pressure was high when she entered the hospital, she had a healthy baby boy.

Other women complained of being unable to hold things in their hands. They dropped utensils when they were cooking. Dr. Ellis gave injections of pyridoxine to one woman who had great difficulty with hands and arms, and edema. He gave her one injection of 50 milligrams of pyridoxine every other day for two weeks. Her edema disappeared along with the painful condition of hands and arms. No mention of salt restriction was made to her. No diuretics were given.

"Edema of pregnancy, long discussed in both medical and lay circles, has become so common," says Dr. Ellis, "that many doctors have come to accept it as being normal during pregnancy, and patients have grown resigned to suffering through it. *It is not normal at all. It is not normal at any time.* The patient feels bad. There is nothing healthy about being swollen with fluids."

The wide disparity of need for pyridoxine in pregnant women is shown in the treatment Dr. Ellis gave his patients. He tells us that he could relieve edema, without diuretics, without salt or fluid restriction, in every woman he treated, by the use of pyridoxine. But varying doses of the vitamin were needed. Two women needed as much as 150 milligrams *by injection* every day. A number needed up to 100 milligrams.

Weight control was related to control of edema. Apparently weight gain was a gain in fluid, nothing more. One nineteen-year-old patient lost 13 pounds in one week after she got 150 milligrams of pyridoxine every day. Another who responded only slightly to 50 milligrams lost 15 pounds in 18 days when she was given 150 milligrams of B_6 daily. Some of the patients were apparently not absorbing the vitamin and had to have it in injections.

The other stories in Dr. Ellis' book are convincing evidence of the usefulness of this B vitamin in pregnancy. In every case the difficulties with edema, numbness, "pins and needles" and other nerve symptoms were alleviated when the dose of vitamin B_6 was high enough.

"If pyridoxine can eliminate edema and assist in halting convulsions—as I believe it will—it is quite possible that the remaining sign, hypertension, could be more easily controlled, and overall mortality of eclampsia could be reduced, if not prevented. It is to be emphasized that the full role of large therapeutic doses of pyridoxine and magnesium in the prenatal period is just beginning to unfold. More investigations in large clinics are needed," says Dr. Ellis.

"In evaluating the fluctuating edema of the hands during pregnancy as well as in the premenstrual period and as a complication of menopausal arthritis," he goes on, "it seems certain that vitamin B_6 deficiency is in some way complicated by an imbalance of steroids (hormones) which is manifested by edema. As mentioned previously, there is laboratory evidence that estrogen, a female hormone, is intimately associated with B_6 metabolism. A sufficient amount of B_6 must be present for proper metabolism of estrogen; otherwise, the patient apparently becomes toxic from estrogen. . . ."

Dr. Ellis concludes this chapter of his book with a summary addressed to physicians who read the book. He states that one may safely give 50 to 450 milligrams of pyridoxine daily and up to 1,000 milligrams daily for short intervals of three to five days during confinement. He says that edema was controlled or prevented by 50 to 450 milligrams of pyridoxine daily in all but six out of 225 of his patients. Numbness and tingling in hands and fingers were relieved by 50 to 450 milligrams of B_6 daily. Inability to hold objects without dropping them was controlled with 50 to 450 milligrams daily. Salt restriction and diuretics were unnecessary for prevention of edema when enough vitamin B_6 was given. Salt was not restricted and water pills were not given to any of the 225 women.

Giving these large doses of B_6 to pregnant women did not result in vitamin B_6 dependency in their babies. That is, the babies did not need any special supplements of the vitamin to be healthy. Large doses of B_6 and magnesium were successful in preventing convulsions in patients with toxemia and eclampsia. Pregnant women with extensive edema of hands, feet and legs lost from 10 to 15 pounds within two weeks when given 50 to 450 milligrams of B_6 daily.

"These conclusions indicate that all pregnant women should have at least 50 milligrams of B_6 as a supplement throughout their pregnancy," says Dr. Ellis, "and many of them should also receive at least 500 milligrams of magnesium daily, and with the appearance of the signs of toxemia the magnesium should be increased to 1,000 milligrams daily."

Dr. Ellis's book was published in 1973. In the intervening five years millions of American women have been taking The Pill. It is now well established that The Pill destroys vitamin B_6 in many women, making their requirements for this vitamin much greater. Certainly women suffering from deficiency in this B vitamin due to The Pill, and then becoming pregnant, have needs for vitamin B_6 that are far greater than women who have not taken The Pill.

CHAPTER 22

Pyridoxine
for Impotence

"ON OCCASION I have found that large dosages of pyridoxine hydrochloride, 50 milligrams twice a day, and cyanocobalamin, 100 micrograms a day, occasionally relieved impotence in patients taking phenelzine. In most cases, however, this regimen was not successful, and if there is no response within two to three weeks, I would suggest an alternate procedure. . . ." said a New York expert in the pages of *The Journal of the American Medical Association* for October 13, 1978.

Pyridoxine is our old friend vitamin B_6. Cyanocobalamin is our old friend vitamin B_{12}. Phenelzine is known in the trade as Nardil, a drug given as an antidepressant and a high blood pressure pill. Joe Graedon in *The Peoples' Pharmacy* tells us that several members of this family of drugs cause impotence. In fact, says Graedon, "drugs which affect the nervous system can occasionally mess up sexual function. . . . Nardil and Parnate have been reported to induce impotence. A depressed patient is not likely to respond favorably to a drug that hinders sexuality. Even common minor tranquilizers, Librium and Valium, can affect sexual desire in some people."

We receive many letters inquiring about remedies for impotence. Never does any correspondent tell us what drugs he is taking, if any. Apparently it seldom occurs to anybody that any drug can mess up many different aspects of life, including sex life. Nicotine, alcohol and caffeine are the drugs used most widely today. Do they cause impotence? Who knows? But if you are worried about impotence why not eliminate these drugs and see if the results are good?

Does the *JAMA* statement indicate that taking vitamin B_6 in quite large doses and taking vitamin B_{12} in quite large doses every day will treat any kind of impotence? Not at all. Even among patients who were taking a drug known to cause impotence, only occasional patients were relieved. But this is no reason not to try the vitamins just in case you are one of the lucky ones who will respond. And there seems no reason to stop after only a few weeks, since these are inexpensive and totally harmless substances.

Pyridoxine is known to be essential for the health of the nervous system. So is vitamin B_{12}. There is startling evidence of the effectiveness of pyridoxine in preventing life-threatening convulsions and other implacable nervous afflictions. Vitamin B_{12} has been used with great success in older folks to treat symptoms of senility. So have other B vitamins. If drugs that affect the nerves may cause impotence, perhaps vitamins that protect the nerves may prevent impotence.

At any rate, it appears that most of us are short on the B vitamins, because of a lifetime of eating refined carbohydrates which contain almost no B vitamins at all and require large amounts of B vitamins for processing in the body's complex mechanisms. So why not add B complex, in rather high potency, to your daily supplements and eat lots of those foods that contain the most B vitamins: the high protein foods including meats, poultry, fish, shellfish, wholegrains, nuts, seeds, legumes, green leafy vegetables and dairy products. Eliminate all drugs, if you possibly can.

CHAPTER 23

Pyridoxine Protects Against Infections

THERE'S GOOD NEWS about two B vitamins in *Medical Tribune* (December 8, 1971)—the news magazine lots of doctors read. A biochemist from the University of Pittsburgh, speaking at a symposium on Nutrition and the Future of Man, said that two B vitamins are essential for the production and transportation in the human body of antibodies—that is, those materials which protect us from infections.

The two vitamins are vitamin B_6 and pantothenic acid, another B vitamin. In any individual who does not have enough of these vitamins in his body, the production of antibodies will be decreased. They will not circulate in the blood to accomplish their biological purpose which is to destroy harmful bacteria.

In addition, lack of pyridoxine tends to make one sensitive to various allergy-producing substances. When animals lack pyridoxine their bodies are inefficient in manufacturing protein and nucleic acids, both of which are essential to life.

When animals lack pantothenic acid, there seems to be a deficiency in the way the body transports proteins from where they are created inside cells to the outside where they are needed.

Why should anybody be concerned these days with de-

Pantothenic Acid Content
of Some Common Foods

(We give the milligram content of one serving, about 100 grams)

Food	Milligrams
Brains (all kinds)	2.6
Broccoli	1.17
Bulgur	0.66
Cabbage juice	1.1
Cashews	1.3
Cauliflower	1
Chicken	1
Chickpeas	1.25
Cottonseed flour	4.32
Eggs, whole	1.6
Filberts	1.14
Flounder	0.85
Heart	3
Kale	1
Kidneys	4
Lentils	1.3
Liver	8
Liverwurst	2.7
Mushrooms	2.2
Oatmeal	1.4
Peanuts	2.8
Peas, dry	2
Rice, Brown	1.1
Salmon	1.3
Sesame seed flour	2.7
Soybeans	1.7
Sunflower seeds	1.4
Turkey	2.67
Walnuts	0.90
Wheat bran	2.9
Wheat germ	1.2
Whey, dried	4
Yeast, brewer's	12

ficiency in these two B vitamins? Both are removed wholesale when flour and cereal products are refined to make commercial products. Neither is returned in the so-called "enrichment" program. Many topnotch experts in the field of nutrition have insisted that pyridoxine must be added to our enriched cereals and breads, foretelling all kinds of nutritional disasters if our baking industry does not take on this added responsibility.

Are you worried about Swine flu, Hong Kong flu or the numerous viruses and infections which plague us from time to time? Have you suffered from recent infections that no amount of antibiotics can handle? Do you have frequent colds? Vitamin C is effective for fighting infections of all kinds.

Dr. Roger J. Williams, a discoverer of the B vitamin pantothenic acid, has shown many times in laboratory experiments at the University of Texas that animals eating a perfectly balanced and highly nutritious diet will live considerably longer and healthier lives if pantothenic acid is added to that already excellent diet.

These experiments are described in Dr. Williams' classic book *Nutrition Against Disease* in which he talks of something he calls "supernutrition"—that is, getting more than one needs of all the vitamins and minerals for super health. This distinguished nutrition expert, who performed more work on vitamins than any other living scientist, believes that the average American is not getting nearly enough pantothenic acid for good health and longevity. Most food supplements do not contain nearly enough of the vitamin to meet the needs of modern human beings, he contends.

Pantothenic acid has been used in treating arthritis. British physicians have found that giving large doses of this B vitamin along with royal jelly (the food bees manufacture to feed their queen) can alleviate arthritis symptoms, if the treatment is continued for quite long periods of time. The blood of arthritis victims has been found to contain almost no pantothenic acid.

Many nutrition experts have warned that pyridoxine at least must be returned to our depleted cereal and bread products if we want to avoid an epidemic of deficiency in this essential nutrient.

Real wholegrain breads and cereals contain all the original pyridoxine and pantothenic acid which was in the original grain. And highly concentrated foods made from these products contain much larger amounts—wheat germ and wheat bran, for example. Other products available at health food stores also contain large amounts. And, of course, B vitamin tablets are available. Supplements of the entire B complex of vitamins are valuable. Good, too, are supplements of the individual ones, from which you can get a higher potency than from the all-in-ones.

The accompanying chart lists those foods which contain pantothenic acid. From the chart you can readily see that the best foods for you and your family are: meats (especially organ meats), fish, poultry, eggs, leafy green vegetables, seed foods like beans, peas, sesame, soybeans, sunflower seeds, plus all those foods made from real wholegrain cereals like brown rice, wholegrain breads and cereals, wheat germ and bran.

We think it is remarkable that a food sold only in health food stores contains more pantothenic acid and pyridoxine than any other foods—brewers yeast. Use it in every food you can slip it into without disturbing the taste—salads, soups, everything you bake like bread, also meatloaves, cereals, granola, fruit juices, milk drinks and so on.

CHAPTER 24

All About Yeast

THAT TINY PACKAGE of greyish powder that you dump into warm water and then stir into your bread dough. That bottle of grayish powder that you dip into and spread over salads and soups. Those grayish tablets that you take with a glass of milk. Can all these really be yeast?

How does it happen, then, that the first powder can be used to raise bread or ferment wine, but that you·don't eat it raw? And how does it happen that the second and third can't be used to raise bread, but can and should be used to improve nutrition? They all look very much alike. What's the difference?

The word Yeast comes from the Sanskrit word *yas* which means "to seethe." Yeast is a microscopic plant which belongs to the family of *Saccharomyces cerevisiae*. These plants are so tiny that they consist of only one cell. In the very early days of human life, our ancestors discovered that if they left fruits or grains in warm moist conditions they changed into intoxicating substances—wine or beer we call them today. The yeast cells from the air or from the skins of the fruit brought about this transformation.

Thousands of years later, human beings had discovered how to plant cereals and were making bread. They usually made it by mixing the ground cereal with a little water, forming a flat cake which they then baked on a hot flat stone.

One day, it seems, a baker forgot and left his dough sitting for a while. When he came back, the dough had swelled until it was double in size. It was light and porous. He put it on the stone to bake and got an entirely new kind of bread— light and airy and much easier and tastier to eat. Some wild yeast in the air had found his bread dough and, because it was warm and moist, the yeast grew, pushing out the dough around its cells. As it grew it gave off carbon dioxide which created bubbles and lightened the dough.

Down through the centuries most bread in Western countries has been "yeasted"—that is, leavened with yeast. In modern days we don't depend on wild yeasts in the air to do the job. We buy baker's yeast and use one or two cakes or packages for our bread-making. Yeast plants grow very rapidly in a process called "budding." From the surface of a cell a small "bud" develops and grows to the size of the parent cell. Then it, too, "buds" and so on. Since this process takes place very rapidly, it is easy to see how a loaf of bread can be leavened in less than an hour, depending on how much baker's yeast you have used and how well you have provided exactly the temperature the yeast needs to grow—70 to 85 degrees or thereabouts.

So baker's yeast can be bought fresh and moist in yeast cakes, which should be kept refrigerated and used rather soon, or powdered in air-tight packages which have a much longer shelf-life. Do not break the seal on these packages until you plan to use the yeast for making bread.

Brewers yeast, food yeast or primary yeast as it may be called, is the same kind of yeast plant except that the plant is inactivated, hence no longer "alive." These are the yeasts you see on the shelves of your health food store. Brewers yeast is the yeast used to make beer, after it has performed its function there and cannot be used again. It is washed free of all alcoholic content and dried. To make beer the yeast is "fed" on a "wort" or mass consisting of grains and/or hops.

Food yeast is also grown on other worts: sugar, corn, potatoes, fruit juice, grain, molasses or waste from several industries. If you are dedicated to the temperance movement there is no need to avoid food yeast because it may have some association with a brewery. It may have been grown, instead, on molasses or grain or fruit juice.

Not so long ago in our South a hideous and mysterious disease ravaged the people. It was pellagra. It brought unsightly skin discolorations, terrible digestive disorders and such serious mental symptoms that its victims went insane. The experts did not know what caused it. After years of fruitless experimentation with drugs and vaccines, several nutrition specialists decided that it might be caused by improper diet. Scientists had found a disease somewhat like it in dogs and had treated the animals successfully with the B vitamin niacin. They gave this to pellagra patients and brought about improvement. But giving them large doses of liver along with all the other members of the B complex of vitamins was even better.

According to Dr. Franklin Bicknell and Dr. Frederick Prescott in *Vitamins in Medicine*, physicians in the 1930's used to treat extremely serious cases of pellagra by giving the patients as much as 100 milligrams of the B vitamin niacin every hour for 10 hours. They would get dramatic improvement in the mental symptoms within a day or so. The digestive and skin conditions took a bit longer. Says Bicknell, "Yeast or other sources of the vitamin B complex such as yeast extract or wheat germ preparations are added to the diet."

Dr. Tom Spies, who got into the fight against pellagra in the early days, used to give his patients as much as half a cup or even a whole cup of brewers yeast every day. This is because brewers yeast is the most abundant source of all the B vitamins, along with many minerals and excellent protein.

Brewers yeast, or food yeast as w
yeast which has been inactivated. Th
themselves are no longer alive. They ca
bread. But the wealth of nutrients, inclu
minerals, which they accumulated while
still there, readily available for human b   use the
yeast.

Gram for Gram,
Wheat Germ and
Brewer's Yeast Are:

Richer in protein than any other food, except gluten flour and several soybean products,

Richer in iron than any other food, except soybean flour and liver,

Richer in magnesium than any other vegetable food, except soybean flour and blackstrap molasses,

Richer in phosphorus than any other food, except squash and pumpkin seeds and powdered milk,

Richer in the B vitamin, thiamine, than any other food, except defatted soybean flour,

Richer in the B vitamin, riboflavin, than any other food, except dried whey, non-fat powdered milk, liver, kidneys,

Richer in the B vitamin, niacin, than any other vegetable food except for certain nuts and beans,

Richer in the B vitamins, pyridoxine and pantothenic acid, than any other vegetable food,

Wheat germ is richer in vitamin E and the healthful unsaturated fats than any other food except for wheat germ oil and other cereal and seed oils.

---

days various names are sometimes given by man-
ers to this kind of yeast. But it is basically all the
me thing, although one yeast may excell in one B vitamin,
others in another B vitamin. And so on. So expert is the
microscopic yeast plant at manufacturing protein and B vitamins that some nutrition experts have proposed growing
food yeast to feed all the hungry people in the undeveloped
countries who lack, chiefly, high-protein food. Protein is
produced very rapidly by the yeast plant. Even a small factory
could turn out relatively enormous amounts of this precious
plant protein, so loaded with B vitamins.

In more recent times still other wondrous substances have
been found in yeast—food yeast. Studying blood sugar disorders, chemists have discovered that the trace mineral chromium helps to stabilize blood sugar, thus helping to prevent
diabetes and its related disorder, low blood sugar or hypoglycemia. They found, too, that a substance which they call
Glucose Tolerance Factor can bring about this improvement,
along with the trace mineral chromium. Glucose Tolerance
Factor is found most abundantly in brewers yeast. Another
excellent reason to use it every day in every way you can
devise.

Why not eat baker's yeast raw? If it's not edible that way
why do we use it to raise bread? Baker's yeast is very edible
and it's also loaded with B vitamins. But in this kind of
yeast, the yeast plants are still very much alive. They need
only warmth and moisture to grow and grow, as they do in
rising bread dough.

Your digestive tract is warm and moist. Eating live yeast
(baker's yeast) forms a yeast factory in your digestive tract
where the yeast goes on growing and reaching out for the B
vitamins and minerals for its own good health. It has to get
these elements somewhere so it robs your digestive tract of
them. This is something you don't want or need. After the
baker's yeast has been baked into bread or rolls however, the

yeast plants are no longer alive and all their wealth of nutrients is available to you in the bread.

Of course you use only a very little bit of yeast for leav-
ening bread. And, generally, you might use only a few ta-
blespoons of brewers yeast in a glass of milk or fruit juice.
Is there enough of the B vitamins there to accomplish anything? You bet there is. Look at the chart on page 155 to
see the comparison between the amount of B vitamins in
brewers yeast and in several foods which are known to be
good sources of B vitamins.

You don't have to take your brewers yeast in milk or fruit
juice, of course. You can add it unobtrusively to almost anything you prepare in the kitchen: soup, salad, casseroles,
breads of all kinds (use the baker's yeast to leaven it and the
brewers yeast to enrich it), mayonnaise and salad dressings,
cereals (cooked or cold), sauces, mashed or creamed vegetables, fruit cocktails, and so on. Any kind of yeast added
to bread improves the taste, for bread is supposed to taste
"yeasty." The taste of brewers yeast added to any of the
above foods may be a bit startling, at first, so do it gradually.
Use only a bit at first, but use it often, in lots of dishes. You
can mix quite large amounts of brewers yeast into peanut
butter without affecting the taste.

There are many classic experiments performed in earlier
days to demonstrate the nutritional excellence of yeast. Perhaps the most astonishing is one of Dr. Clive McCay's at
Cornell University. He put two groups of rats on the same
diet except that one group got five percent brewers yeast in
their food. The rats which got the yeast lived in good health
almost exactly twice as long as those which ate the usual
nourishing laboratory diet without the yeast. Could you want
any better recommendation than that?

Pyridoxine (Vitamin B$_6$)

Pyridoxine is part of the B complex of vitamins. We call it a complex because all of the B vitamins occur in the same foods and work together to provide good nutrition for nerves, skin, brain and digestive tract mostly, although they are also involved in practically everything that goes on inside our bodies.

Pyridoxine (also called vitamin B$_6$) was discovered fairly recently, after scientists found out that the original B vitamin they had discovered was made up of many essential parts. They isolated and named each part and eventually each part was declared officially to be a vitamin, meaning that life and growth for human beings, animals, birds, fish and many smaller forms of life cannot survive without it.

It is well to keep in mind, as you read about the extremely exciting and powerful substance we call pyridoxine, that all the B vitamins work together for good health. It is never wise to take large amounts of one of them and neglect all or most of the others. By eating a highly nourishing diet you can obtain a goodly amount of the B vitamins, including pyridoxine. It is also possible to fortify your diet with supplements of the B vitamins. They are all water soluble, meaning that whatever your body does not need is excreted rather soon, and is not stored to any extent in the body. So you should aim to get plenty of all the B vitamins, including pyridoxine, every day.

Suggested Further Reading

Adams, Ruth, *The Complete Home Guide to All the Vitamins,* Larchmont Books, New York, 1972.

Adams, Ruth, and Frank Murray, *Body, Mind and the B Vitamins,* Larchmont Books, New York, 1972.

Adams, Ruth, and Frank Murray, *Improving Your Health with Vitamin C,* Larchmont Books, New York, 1978.

Adams, Ruth, and Frank Murray, *Improving Your Health with Vitamin E,* Larchmont Books, New York, 1978.

Adams, Ruth, and Frank Murray, *Improving Your Health with Niacin (Vitamin B3),* Larchmont Books, New York, 1978.

Adams, Ruth, and Frank Murray, *Improving Your Health with Zinc,* Larchmont Books, New York, 1978.

Adams, Ruth, and Frank Murray, *Megavitamin Therapy,* Larchmont Books, New York, 1973.

Davis, Adelle, *Let's Get Well,* Harcourt, Brace and World, New York, 1965.

Ellis, John M., M.D., and James Presley, *Vitamin B6, The Doctor's Report,* Harper and Row, New York, 1973.

Hawkins, David, and Linus Pauling, *Orthomolecular Psychiatry,* W. H. Freeman and Company, San Francisco, 1973.

Kaufman, William, *The Common Form of Joint Dysfunction,* Hildreth, 1949. Out of print; see if your library has a copy.

Williams, Roger, *Nutrition Against Disease,* Bantam Books, New York, 1971.

Index

Read What the Experts Say About Larchmont Books!

Body, Mind and the B Vitamins

"I feel that "Body, Mind and the B Vitamins" is an excellent, informative book. I recommend everyone buy two copies; one for home and one to give to their physician."—*Harvey M. Ross, M.D., Los Angeles Calif.*

Program Your Heart for Health

"What is unique about this book is that the tremendous body of fascinating information has been neatly distilled so that the problems and the solutions are quite clear. . . . (This book) will be around for a long time . . . so long as health continues to be the fastest growing failing business in the United States and so long as it is not recognized that the medical problem is not medical but social."—*E. Cheraskin, M.D., D.M.D., Birmingham, Ala.*

"If more people were to read books such as this one and were to institute preventive medical programs early in life, the mortality in heart disease would drop precipitously as well as in our other serious medical problems."—*Irwin Stone, Ph.D., San Jose, Calif.*

"Program Your Heart for Health" contains a wealth of data. I plan to make use of it many times."—*J. Rinse, Ph.D., East Dorset, Vt.*

"This is an important book for your health and well-being." —*Michael Walczak, M.D., Studio City, Calif.*

Read What the Experts Say About Larchmont Books!

Megavitamin Therapy

"This book provides a much-needed perspective about the relationship of an important group of medical and psychiatric conditions, all of which seem to have a common causation (the grossly improper American Diet) and the nutritional techniques which have proven to be of great benefit in their management."—*Robert Atkins, M.D., author of "Dr. Atkins' Diet Revolution," New York.*

"This responsible book gathers together an enormous amount of clinical and scientific data and presents it in a clear and documented way which is understandable to the average reader . . . The authors have provided critical information plus references for the acquisition of even more essential knowledge."—*David R. Hawkins, M.D., The North Nassau Mental Health Center, Manhasset, New York.*

Health Foods

"This book (and "Is Low Blood Sugar Making You a Nutritional Cripple") are companion books worth adding to your library. The fact that one of the books is labeled "health foods" is an indication how far our national diet has drifted away from those ordinary foods to which man has adapted over the past million years. . . ."—*A. Hoffer, M.D., Ph.D., The Huxley Newsletter.*

"A sensible, most enlightening review of foods and their special qualities for maintenance of health. . . ."—*The Homeostasis Quarterly.*

Read What the Experts Say About Larchmont Books!

The Complete Home Guide to All the Vitamins

"This is a handy book to have at home, for it discusses in clear, simple language just what vitamins are, why we need them, and how they function in the body."—*Sweet 'n Low*

"Want to know what vitamins you need and why? Then this is your cup of tea. A paperback that tells you everything you ever wanted to know about vitamins and maybe were afraid to ask . . . Read it and reap."—*Herald American and Call Enterprise, Allentown, Pa.*

Minerals: Kill or Cure?

"Written both for professional and non-professional readers, this book offers excellent background for additional discoveries that are inevitable in the next few years . . ."—*The Total You*

Eating in Eden

"This book contains very valuable information regarding the beneficial effects of eating unrefined foods . . ."—*Benjamin P. Sandler, M.D., Asheville, N.C.*

"We must be reminded again and again what junk (food) does and how much better we would be if we avoided it. This book serves to do this."—*A. Hoffer, M.D., Ph.D.*

"The Complete Home Guide to All the Vitamins"

by Ruth Adams

Foreword by Dr. E. Cheraskin

432 pages $2.95

Have you ever wanted a complete, easy-to-read book on the vitamins and why they are so necessary for good health? In this best-selling book, Ruth Adams gives you in-depth details about Vitamin A, Vitamin B, Vitamin C, Vitamin D, Vitamin E and Vitamin K.

You will learn which foods contain these vitamins and what the recommended daily dietary allowances for each vitamin are. You will also find out what happens when you become deficient in the various vitamins; which vitamins can protect you from pollution and certain food additives; how you can maintain good health if you are eating the right foods and perhaps supplementing your diet with food supplements.

This is a book that should be in every home and every library. Documentation from some of the world's leading authorities on nutrition tells the story: you cannot maintain good health for any length of time if you are not getting these essential vitamins in your diet.

When you do not get these vitamins regularly, something is bound to happen. Find out what in this unusual, timely book.

"Lose Weight, Feel Great!"

by Dr. John Yudkin

220 pages $1.75

Do you want to lose weight but are afraid of the many fad diets that spring up every few months? Do you want to feel slimmer, shed pounds and inches in the right places and look younger?

Then let the internationally famous Dr. John Yudkin of England show you how to lose weight permanently. You do not have to count calories and you do not have to sacrifice good nutrition. There are no tricks, no non-sense, no hunger pangs, no quick weight loss followed by a quick weight gain because you were so hungry you ate everything in sight once you were off your old diet.

The key is in what you eat. Let Dr. Yudkin show you how to count carbohydrate units without counting calories; how to eat the right foods without worrying how much food you are consuming; how to enjoy foods prepared from his tested recipes; how to diet when you are eating in restaurants or at the home of friends; how to diet without losing your cheerful disposition . . . how to stay trim for the rest of your life!

It's fun to look in the mirror and like what you see. "Lose Weight, Feel Great" just may be the book that will help that dream come true.

"Minerals: Kill or Cure?"

by Ruth Adams and Frank Murray

Foreword by Dr. Harvey M. Ross

378 pages $1.95

In this exceptional book, Adams and Murray tell you all about the minerals and trace minerals: the ones you need everyday for optimum nutrition and the ones that can endanger your life.

In the most complete book on the subject for the layman, you will read complete, in-depth chapters on: Calcium, Phosphorus, Iodine, Iron, Magnesium, Zinc, Sodium, Potassium, Chloride, Copper, Chromium, Cobalt, Manganese, Molybdenum, Selenium, Lithium, Fluoride, Beryllium, Nickel, Cadmium, Vanadium, Mercury, Lead and information about many of the lesser-known trace elements (Antimony, Arsenic, Barium, Bismuth, Boron, Silicon, Silver, Sulfur, Tin, Uranium, Zirconium, etc.)

You will learn hundreds of startling facts about minerals: doctors often diagnose heart attacks by the amount of manganese in the body; chromium, magnesium, manganese and vitamin B6 deficiency are related to diabetes; kelp contains over 26 trace minerals; mercury can kill unborn children; many baby foods contain too much sodium; lead is linked to multiple sclerosis; etc.

"Megavitamin Therapy"

by Ruth Adams and Frank Murray

Foreword by Dr. David Hawkins

Introduction by Dr. Abram Hoffer

280 pages $1.95

This is one of the most exciting books on health and nutrition that you may ever read. It is the first and most complete book on the subject, with over 100,000 copies in print.

There is considerable evidence—and Adams and Murray spell this out in detail in the book—that alcoholism, schizophrenia (a major mental illness), hyperactivity in children and even drug addiction are often the result of a lifelong improper diet. After a person has been eating incorrectly for many years, certain deficiencies and forms of malnutrition begin to appear. One of the causes may also be low blood sugar.

To correct these deficiencies and to return the patient to boundless good health, many physicians and psychiatrists are turning to megavitamin therapy. They do this with a corrective diet and massive doses of certain vitamins. After years of neglect, it may take the body some time to correct itself.

But these disorders can be controlled, as you will learn in this fascinating book. Many case histories tell the story.

*The best books on health
and nutrition are from*

LARCHMONT BOOKS

Almonds to Zoybeans, by 'Mothey' Parsons, 192 pages, $1.50.

Arthritis, by Adams and Murray, 256 pages, $2.25.

Beverages, by Adams and Murray, 286 pages, $1.75.

Body, Mind and the B Vitamins, by Adams and Murray, Foreword by Dr. Abram Hoffer, 320 pages, $1.95.

The Compleat Herbal, by Ben Charles Harris, 352 pages, $1.95.

The Complete Home Guide to All the Vitamins, by Ruth Adams, Foreword by E. Cheraskin, M.D., 432 pages, $2.95.

Eating in Eden, by Ruth Adams, 196 pages, $1.75.

Fighting Depression, by Harvey M. Ross, M.D., 224 pages, $1.95.

Food for Beauty, by Helena Rubenstein, Revised and Updated by Frank Murray, 256 pages, $1.95.

The Good Seeds, the Rich Grains, the Hardy Nuts, for a Healthier Life, by Adams and Murray, Foreword by Dr. Neil Stamford Painter, 304 pages, $1.75.

Health Foods, by Adams and Murray, Foreword by Dr. S. Marshall Fram, 352 pages, $2.50.

How to Control Your Allergies, by Robert Forman; Ph.D., Foreword by Marshall Mandell, M.D., 256 pages, $1.95.

Is Low Blood Sugar Making You a Nutritional Cripple? by Adams and Murray, Introduction by Robert C. Atkins, M.D., 176 pages, $1.75.

Lose Weight, Feel Great!, by John Yudkin, M.D., Ph.D., 224 pages, $1.75.

Megavitamin Therapy, by Adams and Murray, Foreword by Dr. David Hawkins, Introduction by Dr. Abram Hoffer, 288 pages, $1.95.

Minerals: Kill or Cure? by Adams and Murray, Foreword by Dr. Harvey M. Ross, 368 pages, $1.95.

The New High Fiber Diet, by Adams and Murray, 320 pages, $2.25.

Program Your Heart for Health, by Frank Murray, Foreword by Michael Walczak, M.D., Introduction by E. Cheraskin, M.D., 368 pages, $2.95.